Teen Guide to HEALTH AND WELLNESS

Gail Snyder

ReferencePoint Press

San Diego, CA

About the Author

Gail Snyder is a freelance writer and advertising copywriter who has written twenty-five books for young readers. She lives in Chalfont, Pennsylvania, with her husband, Hal Marcovitz.

Printed in the United States

For more information, contact:
ReferencePoint Press, Inc.
PO Box 27779
San Diego, CA 92198
www.ReferencePointPress.com

Picture Credits:
Cover: Shutterstock.com

6: FatCamera/iStock
10: SDI Productions/iStock
14: New Africa/Shutterstock
18: Schimbator Studio/Shutterstock
23: Creativa Images/Shutterstock
27: Maury Aaseng
29: Mateg Kastlic/Shutterstock
31: PeopleImages/Shutterstock
35: gowithstock/Shutterstock
39: Demkat/Shutterstock
43: Maury Aaseng
45: Akarawut/Shutterstock
47: PonyWang/iStock
50: Prostock-studio/Shutterstock
51: tumka vodka/Shutterstock
54: Pixel-Shot/Shutterstock

LIBRARY OF CONGRESS CATALOGING-IN-PUBLICATION DATA

Name: Snyder, Gail- author
Title: Teen Guide to Health and Wellness/by Gail Snyder
Description: San Diego, CA: ReferencePoint Press, Inc, 2027.
| Includes bibliographical references and index.
Identifiers: LCCN 2026000030 (print) | ISBN
9781678213688 library binding | ISBN 9781678213695 ebook
Subjects: LCSH: Juvenile literature

For compete cataloging-in-publication data please go to www.loc.gov.

CONTENTS

Choosing Wellness

Sixteen-year-old Julia Weissman spends a lot of time thinking about living a healthy lifestyle and sharing information she finds interesting with other teens through an online community called Peer Health Exchange. The exchange is a national nonprofit that helps teens make healthy decisions. Along the way, Weissman has learned how to recognize health tips that sound too good to be true and even dangerous. She says, "As a teen myself, I've experienced firsthand how easy it is to stumble upon unreliable health information. From strange 'home remedies' that suggest putting potatoes in your socks to cure a cold, to more serious misinformation like anti-vaccination movements that spread fear and confusion, it's all out there. And the danger is real."[1]

> "As a teen myself, I've experienced firsthand how easy it is to stumble upon unreliable health information. From strange 'home remedies' that suggest putting potatoes in your socks to cure a cold, to more serious misinformation like anti-vaccination movements that spread fear and confusion, it's all out there."[1]
>
> —Julia Weissman, age sixteen

Social media, she has learned, is a common source of misinformation, and users need to approach it with a healthy dose of skepticism. She adds:

> Social media is filled with oversimplified advice that claims conditions like anxiety or depression can be solved by "thinking positively" or just exercising, which can discourage teens from seeking the professional help they truly need. In sex education, myths about contraception, STIs [sexually transmitted infections], and consent circulate widely, leading to misunderstandings that can result in risky behaviors and misinformed choices. Fitness trends also in-

troduce misinformation through extreme diets, "quick fix" workout routines, and detoxes that promise drastic results but often ignore the needs of growing bodies, potentially causing long-term health issues. Across these domains, misinformation can have long-lasting impacts on teens' physical, mental, and emotional well-being.[2]

Weissman has adopted some guidelines that help her separate evidence-based health information from faddish or harmful advice. For example, she advises being skeptical about advice that doesn't come from well-respected websites like WebMD or the Mayo Clinic. WebMD's articles are written by physicians or medical journalists for an audience that includes consumers, physicians, and health care professionals. The Mayo Clinic is a 150-year-old not-for-profit hospital headquartered in Rochester, Minnesota, with offices worldwide. Weissman suggests teens ask themselves whether the advice seems too simple or makes unrealistic promises. And she gives more weight to advice that cites medical studies that can be checked.

Choosing Wellness

Like Weissman, teens who want to feel their best and function at their highest levels need to understand the concepts of health and wellness. Think of them as fraternal twins—related yet different—who go everywhere together. Health is the physical twin. Weight, height, and a tendency to sneeze during pollen season are some aspects of health. Wellness is the very active twin, representing the choices teens continually make on what they eat or how much sleep they get. The wellness choices teens make affect their mind, mood, relationships, and physical health.

The good news is that teens can decide to make changes to their lifestyles and, in doing so, may avoid the perils affecting their generation. Those perils include a mental health crisis, with soaring anxiety and depression rates. Teens who have anxiety spend much of their lives feeling worried and fearful, while depressed teens may be sad, feel listless, have trouble sleeping or getting out of bed, and think about harming themselves.

By prioritizing wellness, individual teens can move the needle toward improving their concentration in school and avoiding accidents, injuries, and serious health problems such as obesity, heart disease, loneliness, and addiction. Teens who find themselves heading in a direction they don't like might feel stuck. The good thing about being young is that there is plenty of time to make changes. The key is to go slowly.

Positive changes can be made thoughtfully and gradually. "Don't expect to change your eating, drinking, physical activity, or sleeping habits overnight. Changing too much too fast may limit

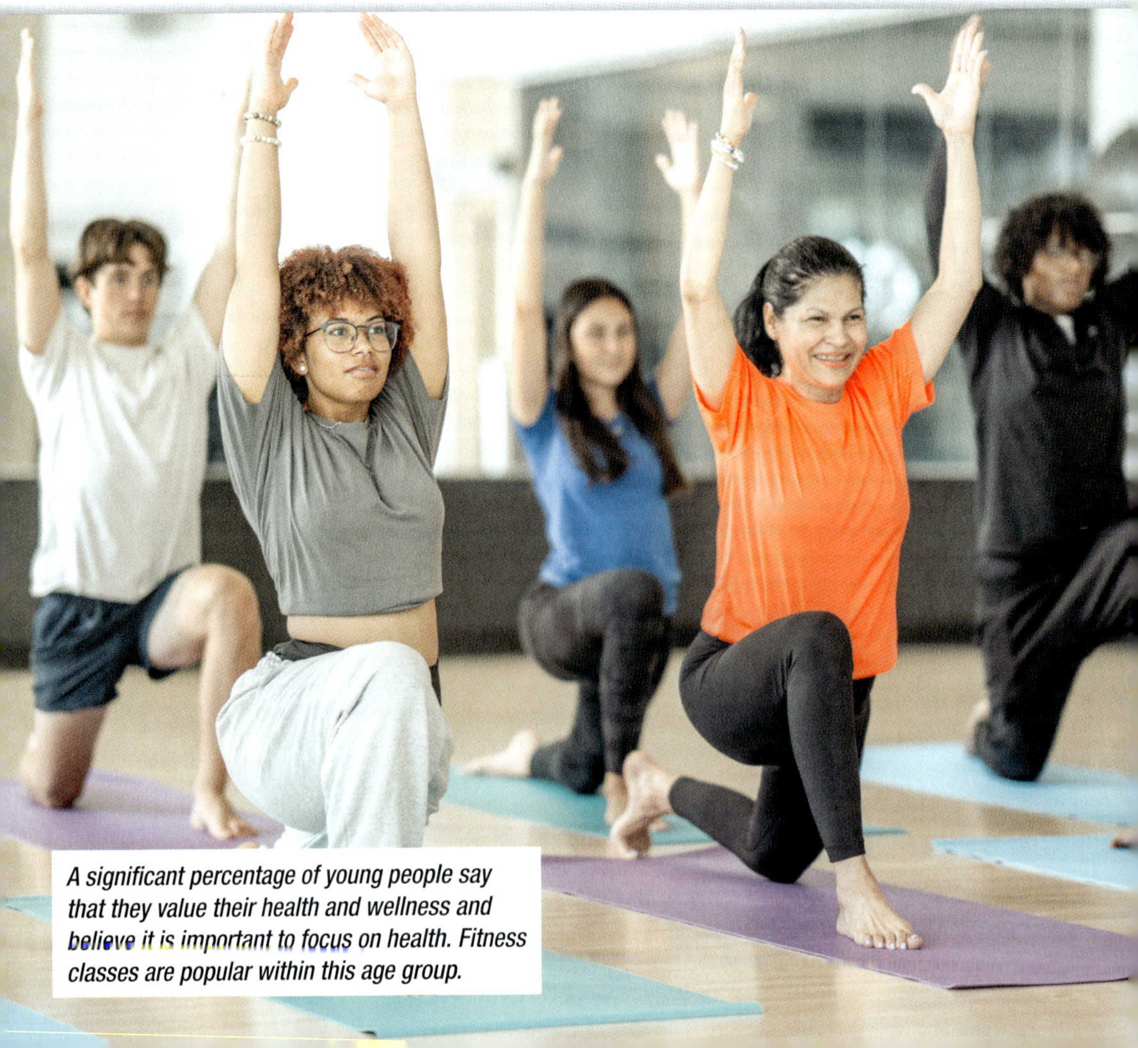

A significant percentage of young people say that they value their health and wellness and believe it is important to focus on health. Fitness classes are popular within this age group.

your chances of success,"[3] advises the National Institute of Diabetes and Digestive and Kidney Diseases, a government agency that disseminates health information as part of the National Institutes of Health.

Technology Has a Positive Role Too

Of course, having health advice at one's fingertips—especially with the proper skepticism—can also be a positive thing. In fact, it may explain why the oldest members of Generation Z (those born from 1997 to 2012) seem to have an appetite for everything health related. McKinsey & Company, a New York City–based international marketing research company that helps identify trends for its clients, says it believes that Gen Z's greater access to health information at younger ages is at least partially to account for its embrace of fitness. In a recent report, the market research company said 56 percent of older Gen Z members rate being fit as important, compared to only 40 percent of all US consumers. For example, fitness classes and gyms are popular among young people.

> "Don't expect to change your eating, drinking, physical activity, or sleeping habits overnight. Changing too much too fast may limit your chances of success."[3]
>
> —National Institute of Diabetes and Digestive and Kidney Diseases

These young adults are telling marketers that they value health and fitness and are willing to pay for products and services that help them achieve their goals. Perhaps their younger brothers and sisters will do the same when they leave their teenage years.

CHAPTER ONE

Teens and the Challenges of Mental Health

Cady had always been a model student. In addition to earning good grades, she was a talented musician and enthusiastic actor in school plays while aspiring to a career in video game design. But when she started a new middle school at age fourteen, the Wisconsin teen knew something wasn't right. She was experiencing worries she could not identify.

Cady found herself troubled by her moods, decision-making abilities, and coping skills—all of which can be challenging for many young people as they move from childhood to adolescence. During this developmental period, teens often experience greater stress as they feel more pressure to get good grades and participate in more extracurricular activities. They may also be more aware of family problems such as tensions between their parents. And all of that is happening at a time when their hormones—the chemical messengers associated with growth, puberty, and well-being—are fluctuating and leaving them emotionally vulnerable.

Cady's pediatrician knew that teens are prone to experiencing stresses on their mental health known as anxiety and depression. During an annual checkup with her doctor, Cady acknowledged experiencing more than the usual level of anxiety, an emotion that typically expresses itself as fear, apprehension, or unease about common events in everyday life. Cady's anxiety often caused feelings of dread and a sick feeling in her stomach. But as she learned more about her own mental health, she found there is no reason to feel embarrassed about having anxiety. She says, "People with anxiety might be feeling bad or stressed not because there's something wrong with them, but just because it's just a condition they have."[4]

> "People with anxiety might be feeling bad or stressed not because there's something wrong with them, but just because it's just a condition they have."[4]
>
> —Cady, a teenager

Treating Anxiety and Depression

With Cady's problem identified, her doctor helped Cady's family find a therapist she could talk to about her feelings. Talk therapy encourages people to share their emotions with a professional who can then suggest better ways to handle them. "It's good to have someone you trust who knows what they're doing. It's been instrumental for me in changing the way I deal with my anxiety," Cady says. "When I'm in a stressful situation, I can say to myself, 'This is just my anxiety, it's going to be okay.'"[5]

One of the techniques her therapist taught her involves what to say to herself when anxious thoughts appear. For example, if she is worried about an upcoming test, she might remind herself, "I am a good student, how I do on this test is not going to make or break me, and I can always do better on the next assignment." Having these prompts can change a student's perspective from a feeling of dread to anticipation that things will go well.

In addition to talk therapy, some teens may also be prescribed a medication to take the edge off their anxiety. Typically, they are prescribed drugs known as serotonin reuptake inhibitors (SSRIs). Taken every day or during an anxiety episode, SSRIs work by increasing the amount of serotonin, a mood-regulating hormone, in a person's brain. In other words, serotonin helps promote positive thoughts, emotional stability, and a relaxing attitude. Commonly prescribed SSRI drugs include Zoloft and Prozac, which often reduce feelings of anxiety within a few weeks.

SSRIs are also effective in treating depression—another common mental condition that may result in constant feelings of sadness, hopelessness, despair, and a loss of interest in participating

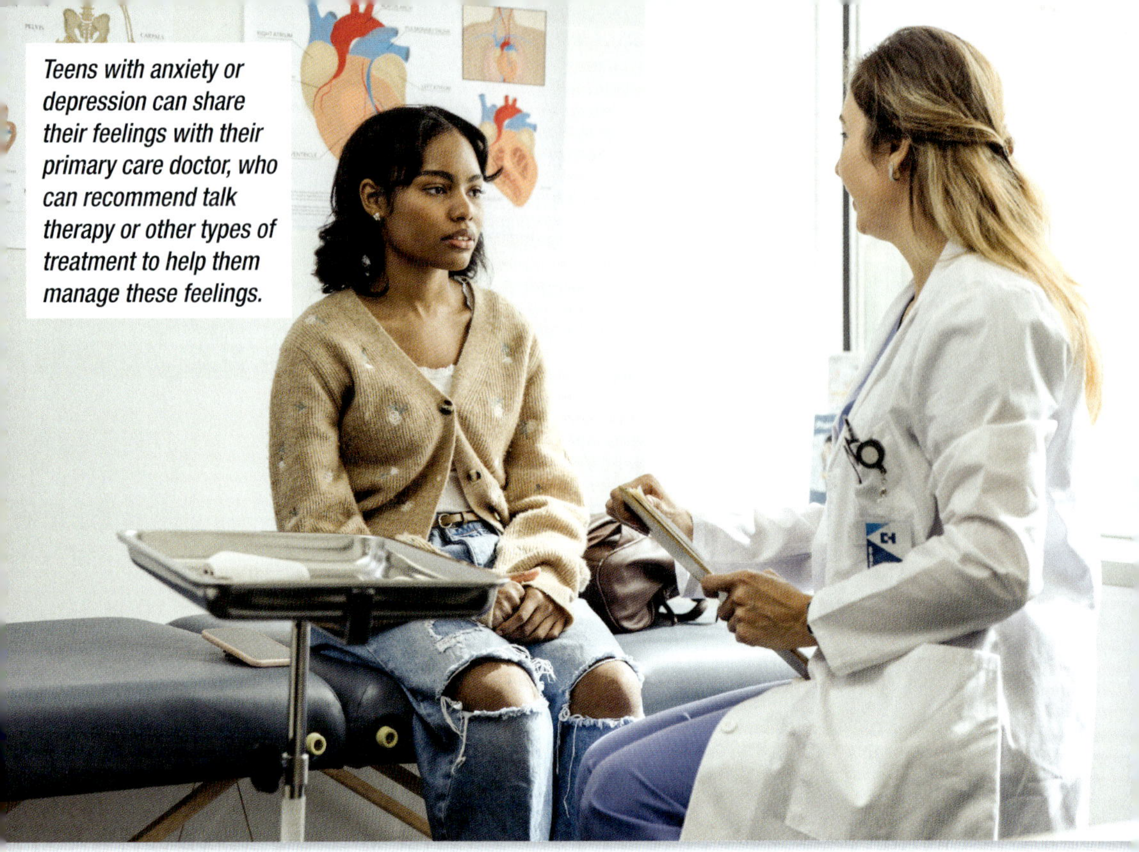

Teens with anxiety or depression can share their feelings with their primary care doctor, who can recommend talk therapy or other types of treatment to help them manage these feelings.

in typical activities such as meeting up with friends, attending to schoolwork, or pursuing hobbies. Depression is a common mental health issue among teenagers. In fact, in 2022 when the Centers for Disease Control and Prevention (CDC)—a federal agency that helps guide national health policies—surveyed high school students, 44 percent said they had recently felt sad or hopeless. Persistent feelings of hopelessness can happen to anyone. Some teens may be more prone to them due to a family history of the illness; others may develop depression after living through traumatic events.

Seventeen-year-old Isaac Rivera of Denver, Colorado, knows that he is not to blame for having depressive symptoms. He says:

> Depression isn't much of a choice. It's different for everyone, and often we can't face it alone—and it's why we're scared to ask for help. . . . I was one of the lucky ones. I asked for help when I knew I couldn't control who I was

> anymore. The scariest thing about depression is that it's you. It's an illness inside your head that is as real as you and me. The moment I took it all in, that moment that I accepted help and realized what I had become, that was the moment the healing could start.[6]

Severe depression can also lead to thoughts of self-harm—including a desire to commit suicide. According to a 2021 CDC study, each year some two thousand young people in America ages fourteen to eighteen take their own lives—and depression is seen as a major cause. An earlier study, performed by psychologists at the University of California, Los Angeles, reported, "Depression, which is also a serious problem for adolescents, is the most significant biological and psychological risk factor for teen suicide."[7]

"Depression isn't much of a choice. It's different for everyone, and often we can't face it alone—and it's why we're scared to ask for help."[6]

—Isaac Rivera, age seventeen

Stephen Satterfield, an eighteen-year-old from Grand Junction, Colorado, fell into a fit of depression and believes telling a friend about his depressive feelings helped save his life. He urges other teens who are thinking about suicide to reach out to a friend, family member, teacher, or suicide prevention hotline—a service often provided by city or state governments. He says:

> When I was 10 minutes away from ending it all, my best friend Kyler called me to see what was going on and we started talking about my problems. Kyler proved to me that people love me and care about me. . . . Everything he told me that night was true. People do care about you, especially your friends and family. They deserve to know what is going on in your head so they can help you. No matter how hard it is, there is always someone there for you willing to listen and help you work through your problems.[8]

Social Media: Good or Bad?

Over the past few years, many teens experiencing anxiety and depression have been able to connect with friends through social media—and since friends can often be the go-to source to help teens overcome their feelings of anxiety and depression, social media platforms can be a way for troubled teens to find relief. According to the Pew Research Center, a well-known organization that designs surveys to solicit opinions on various issues, 74 percent of the teens it contacted reported that social media allows them to feel closer to their friends. In the same survey, just 52 percent of teens felt comfortable raising mental health issues with their parents. As for teachers, more than half of the

Chatbots Can Affect Mental Health in Teens

Many teens are increasingly trying out online companions called chatbots—computer programs that use artificial intelligence, or AI, to engage in dialogue that can seem so realistic many users may forget they are not communicating with real people. A July 2025 survey by Common Sense Media—a resource that recommends books, publications, movies, TV shows, and websites that are not harmful to mental health—found that 72 percent of teens have used chatbots, with 12.5 percent specifically doing so for mental health advice. But chatbots are not trained mental health professionals—the information they provide to users is gleaned from sources found on the internet. Many of those sources may not provide accurate or valuable information. Some experts have already blamed chatbots for leading to harm for teens who discussed ending their lives with them.

Teens would do well to avoid turning to chatbots when they are feeling isolated, because these artificial companions can make those problems worse. Nina Vasan, a professor of psychiatry at Stanford University in California, recommends that teenagers not use AI until more safeguards are put in place to ensure they are not given harmful advice. Says Vasan, "Teens might use these AI systems to avoid real-world social challenges, increasing their isolation rather than reducing it."

Quoted in John Sanford, "Why AI Companions and Young People Can Make for a Dangerous Mix," Stanford Medicine, August 27, 2025. https://med.stanford.edu.

surveyed teens said they would not bring their problems to the attention of their teachers.

Some 34 percent of teens said they at least occasionally get mental health insights from TikTok as well as other platforms, and an even more impressive 63 percent said social media is a good place to get information about their mental health. But while social media can be a place where teens can connect with friends who can help them overcome their feelings of anxiety and depression, social media can also make matters worse. While on social media, many teens find themselves the victims of cyberbullies. These are people teens encounter online who repeatedly say harmful things about them (whether true or not), call them names, ridicule them, and make them feel small, isolated, humiliated, and powerless. But here, too, teens should not suffer in silence, because there are ways to stop the bullies—including bullies they encounter in real life. Methods for dealing with bullies differ depending on whether the bullying is face-to-face or online. But in both cases, telling an adult about the bullying is advisable.

Stopping Bullies

Cyberbullying is an ordeal experienced by about a third of fifty-seven hundred middle and high school students surveyed by the Florida-based Cyberbullying Research Center, which was established to study cyberbullying and advise young people on how to respond to such attacks. According to the organization, locking out and otherwise ignoring the cyberbullies are the most common strategies for halting the behavior. Bullies are found to get satisfaction out of exchanges with the people they target. And so, when their targets ignore or block them, they eventually lose interest and move on to other victims.

A twelve-year-old boy who lives in Arkansas did tell his parents about his encounters with cyberbullying. "My dad showed me how to block the person on Facebook and how to block them on my phone," says the boy. "He also phoned the person's

> "My dad showed me how to block the person on Facebook and how to block them on my phone. He also phoned the person's parents and told them if it happened again, he would phone the police."[9]
>
> —Anonymous twelve-year-old

parents and told them if it happened again, he would phone the police."[9] The Cyberbullying Research Center also recommends that teens report bullies to the social media platform they are using and taking photos or screenshots of the abusive posts to offer as proof.

As for teens who find themselves the victims of bullying at school, the basketball court, skateboard park, or anywhere else they may be spending time, there are solutions for them as well. Teens who are bullied at school can certainly report their bullies to teachers. But friends and other students may step up in their defense as well.

Finding Strength

Lily is an otherwise shy teen who noticed that a classmate whom she did not know very well was the victim of bullying by a teen named Marcus and his friends. Marcus enjoyed taking the class-

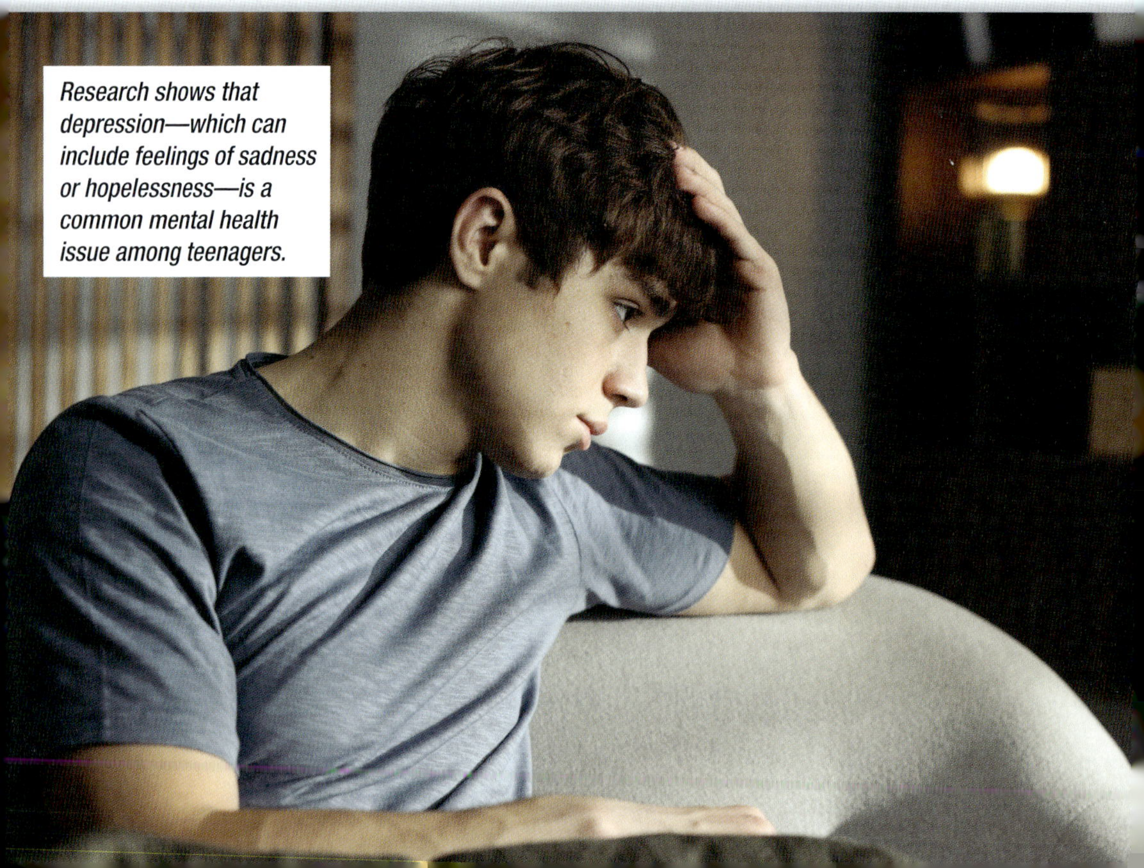

Research shows that depression—which can include feelings of sadness or hopelessness—is a common mental health issue among teenagers.

Teens' Biggest Worries

As a group, teens are worriers. But what do they worry about most, and what can they do about it? Newport Academy, a provider of behavioral health care for teenagers, offers some answers. According to the academy, teens worry most about getting good grades and getting into college, their mental health, body image issues, romantic relationships (or the lack of them), bullying, being labeled a failure, whether they will do well in college or in their careers, and what will happen to the world around them. The latter includes things such as worries about climate change and gun violence.

While a certain amount of worry is normal, teens who would like to worry less can benefit from some strategies. When unwanted concerns arise, teens can shift their focus to something positive, such as finding three things that went well that day and how they helped bring those things about. Other ways to focus less on what bothers teens are taking time to practice a hobby or sport and writing in a journal kept for the purpose of recording worrisome thoughts.

mate's backpack and shoving him into school lockers. Lily found it within herself to speak up in defense of her classmate. She confronted Marcus, telling him to return her classmate's backpack and stop bullying him or she would report Marcus and his friends to a teacher. Marcus backed off, and Lily found a new friend in the classmate who had been bullied. Says the formerly bullied teen, "Marcus still gave me dirty looks, but he didn't touch my backpack again. And I found a new kind of strength, not in fighting back, but in knowing that I wasn't alone. . . . I also had a friend, and a little bit of my old courage back."[10]

Teens should be aware that mental health problems can affect anyone and that seeking help is a sign of strength rather than weakness. If teens believe they are experiencing anxiety or depression, they would do well to share their concern with their family doctor, their parents, a school counselor, or a friend. As Cady demonstrated, teens can lead full lives even as they cope with mental health challenges using the tools they are taught.

CHAPTER TWO

Teens and Sex

When Marija was a teenager, she decided that she would practice abstinence—or refrain from sexual relationships—until marriage. It is a choice she remains happy with even in her early twenties. She says:

> When I was in high school, I saw a lot of my friends go through bad breakups. I watched them worry all the time about getting pregnant or an STI. Both of my brothers became teen dads at a young age. I saw how much it changed their lives; paying child support, visitations, and dealing with ex-girlfriends. Seeing all of this . . . made me decide that I was not going to be like them. I was only going to have sex or even be physically active with one person, and that person was going to be my husband. . . . I can go to bed each night and not wonder if I'm pregnant or have an STI.[11]

Many young people wrestle with the question of whether to engage in a sexual relationship while still in their teen years and, beyond that, prior to their wedding night. As Marija's decision illustrates, some teens choose abstinence. But other teens decide they are ready and willing to engage in sexual relationships. In either case, it is a good idea for teens to know more about what constitutes a healthy relationship, how to communicate their wishes to another person, and even how to tell whether another person has consented to sexual activity. They will also want to know how to protect themselves from pregnancy and STIs.

Ready or Not?

The teenage years are full of curiosity and openness to new experiences, both lending themselves to sexual exploration. But some teens are more mature than others physically, mentally, and emotionally. So, how do teens know whether they are ready for the responsibilities of being sexually active?

> "Both of my brothers became teen dads at a young age. I saw how much it changed their lives; paying child support, visitations, and dealing with ex-girlfriends. Seeing all of this . . . made me decide that I was not going to be like them."[11]
>
> —Marija, a teenager

The answer is by gathering information and looking within themselves to figure out what is important to them and what they are willing to risk. Some teens are focused on getting good grades, playing sports, and working in after-school jobs. They have sexual urges like everyone else but may want to wait until they are older and more mature before acting on them. Dave is like that. He decided he was not ready to have sex as a teen and to save the experience for a woman with whom he would share a true emotional attachment. He says, "I know that sex is great and that my virginity is something I can only give once so I don't want to waste it on just some girl."[12]

In the meantime, he might find himself having to say no to sex clearly and confidently. And that takes practice. Of course, teens who share Dave's beliefs need to be honest without hurting the other person's feelings. A young person out on a date might say, "I'm having a good time, and I like you, but I don't want to have sex until I am older." Or "I plan to wait until I am married to have sex." To avoid potentially awkward moments, young people can create dates where other couples are present.

While young people may have reasons for avoiding sex, there are certainly many other teens who are anxious for the experience of a sexual relationship. Planned Parenthood, the nation's leading provider of reproductive health care services, suggests these teens take stock of their reasons. For example, if they are thinking about having sex because their boyfriend or girlfriend has

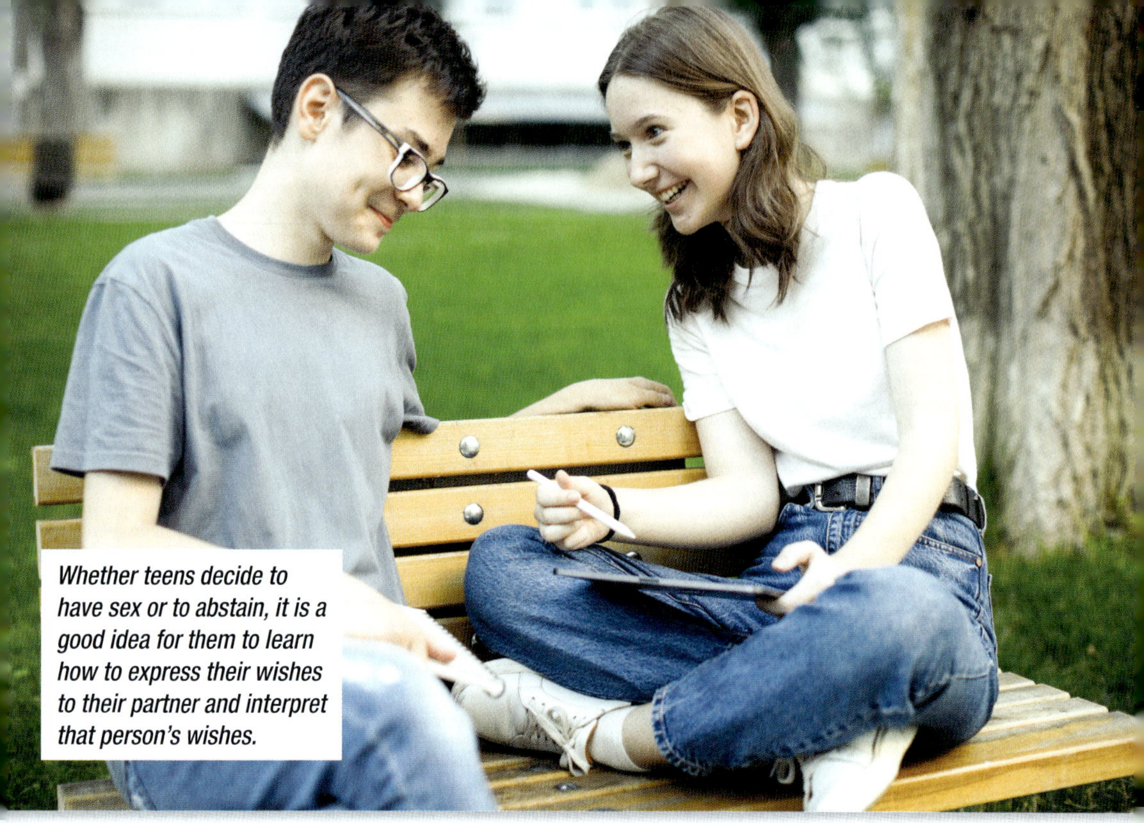

Whether teens decide to have sex or to abstain, it is a good idea for them to learn how to express their wishes to their partner and interpret that person's wishes.

threatened to break up with them if they refuse to begin a sexual relationship, they are better off breaking up—painful as it might be. If young people believe that being sexually active is their ticket to greater popularity among their peers, it is not. Sexual experiences could lead to feelings of regret. And if young people have reached the conclusion that they are the only ones among their friends not having sex, they are probably wrong: The average age at which people first have sex has been climbing and is now over seventeen, according to the CDC.

Spotting Red Flags

Teens should not feel bad about refusing to engage in sex even if that means avoiding relationships with people who are jealous, who try to isolate them, or who make unreasonable demands and prey on their emotions. The boyfriends and girlfriends may at first seem charming, but their nagging insistence on having sex when their partners aren't ready may lead to rocky relationships and ultimately breakups.

Couples who respect each other don't put their own needs ahead of their partner. They make joint decisions based on frank discussions, and they desire to protect each other from harm. These are the couples best equipped to consider the consequences that sexual activity can lead to, such as unwanted pregnancies and STIs. For these couples, who recognize that having unprotected sex is irresponsible, practicing birth control is a shared responsibility.

Discussing Birth Control

Couples seeking options for preventing pregnancy have many from which to choose. For example, oral contraceptives (more commonly known as birth control pills) are an effective and popular means of preventing pregnancy for adolescents. They come

Understanding Consent

Requesting and receiving permission before doing anything sexual with another person is vital. But sometimes people struggle with the concept. The nonprofit health advocacy group Planned Parenthood states that consent must be freely given, reversible, informed, and specific. One who has previously had sex with an individual can decide not to do so again, can decide exactly what they are willing and not willing to do in bed, and must not be coerced, forced, or intimidated. People who are intoxicated or high on drugs are incapable of giving consent because they are impaired. Across the United States and in many other countries, engaging in sex with someone without the partner's consent is regarded as a serious crime.

One anonymous sixteen-year-old girl thought she had adequately signaled to her boyfriend that he was going too far, but he didn't get the message or wasn't listening. Afterward she realized she had not been specific. She never said no. "I thought it was okay, like, I was saying, 'Hey, you got to slow down there.' But," she says, "it didn't come out that way. Then stupid sex just kind of happened." Clear communication is important to ensure that everyone is on the same page.

Quoted in Terri Apter, "What Do Teens Today Understand About Sex and Consent?," Well Doing, May 23, 2022. https://welldoing.org.

in two forms, those prescribed by physicians and those available without a prescription for purchase online and in drugstores and pharmacies.

Physicians often prescribe pills that combine progesterone and estrogen, two natural hormones that can interfere with the teen's menstrual cycle. They are effective at preventing pregnancy 92 percent of the time and do not affect a teen's future ability to get pregnant. The pills must be taken every day. Their cost may be covered by the teen's health insurance plan. Depending on the state the teen lives in, parental consent may be required before a physician can prescribe the pills.

Opill is the name of the over-the-counter birth control pill that can be purchased without a doctor's visit. It works by releasing a synthetic hormone that makes it more difficult for sperm to fertilize an egg. The Opill is 98 percent effective at preventing conception. A month's supply currently costs about $20, or about $240 a year.

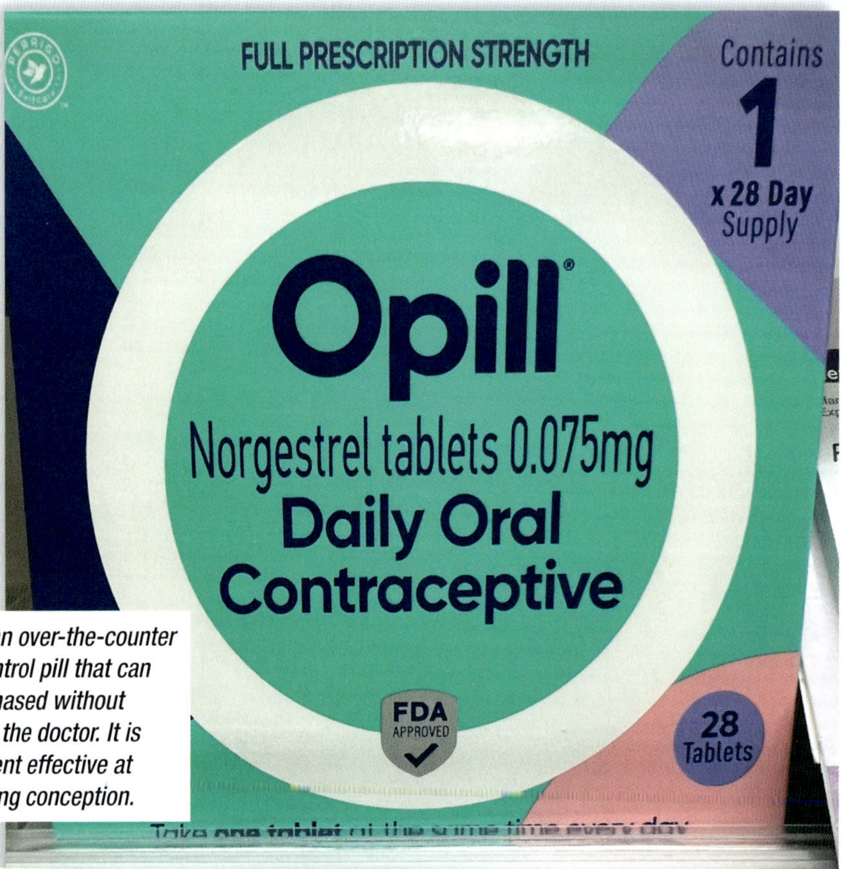

Opill is an over-the-counter birth control pill that can be purchased without going to the doctor. It is 98 percent effective at preventing conception.

IUDs, Implants, and Condoms

There are also options for teens who do not want to take pills. Intrauterine devices (IUDs) and birth control implants are reversible, largely side effect–free, and take care of a young woman's birth control needs for at least three years. For these reasons, Dr. Nicole W. Karjane, a gynecologist, frequently asks her teenage patients to consider these methods of birth control.

An IUD is inserted during a pelvic examination in which the patient, naked from the waist down, lays back on an examination table, placing their feet in stirrups. The stirrups make it easy for the doctor to access the patient's uterus, the expandable abdominal organ in which a fetus grows. IUDs work by releasing a hormone that prevents the release of an egg that can be fertilized. (Some IUDs discharge a small amount of copper into the uterus to impede egg fertilization.)

Birth control implants are inserted under the skin of a girl's forearm after a topical anesthetic is used to numb the area. The process takes about ten minutes, and no pelvic exam is needed. Birth control implants introduce a steady stream of a pregnancy-blocking hormone into a teen's bloodstream.

While most birth control options are designed for women, there is one method for men that Karjane says all sexually active teens should be using: the condom. Condoms, which are often made of a rubberlike substance called latex, are worn over an erect penis. When used correctly, they are up to 98 percent effective at preventing pregnancy. They can be discreetly purchased via drugstores, online vendors, supermarkets, and bodegas, making them convenient and affordable contraceptives. In addition, they are useful for preventing sexually transmitted infections, which is why Karjane recommends that any sexually active teen use them as an adjunct to any other type of contraceptive they may use. Still, condoms are only useful if they are worn each time a couple has intercourse, which is why additional birth control methods may be desirable.

A Pregnant Teen's Story

Izzy Nelsen was sixteen years old when she met her boyfriend. About a year later, they began having sex. But then the unexpected happened. Izzy became pregnant. Her boyfriend broke up with her, and Izzy had some big decisions to make: Should she have an abortion, give her baby up for adoption, or raise the baby as a single teenage mother? After many months of crying and agonizing, she decided to have the baby and raise him.

Fortunately, she had the support of her parents and their church. Members of the church outfitted the young mother with many of the goods she needed to take care of a newborn. Even so, the pregnancy was difficult, and as much as she loves her young son Jonah, she does not recommend that other teens follow in her footsteps. "I wouldn't recommend teen pregnancy to anyone. It was a hard path; it wasn't glamorous at all," she says.

As a teenage parent, Izzy is far from alone, although statistics suggest that fewer teens are giving birth. The Centers for Disease Control and Prevention says the teen birth rate plunged nearly 80 percent from 1991 to 2021. And the decline appears to be ongoing.

Quoted in Trizzy, *Pregnant at 17: My Teen Pregnancy Story*, YouTube, June 2, 2024. www.youtube.com/watch?v=t-trs9QP9DA.

Gaining Knowledge

It is important for teenagers to learn about contraceptives and how they work because many teenagers harbor misconceptions about them. That's what pediatric emergency medicine physician Cynthia Mollen learned after seeing teenagers who have come to her emergency room for various injuries or illnesses. Many seventeen-year-old girls she has met in emergency rooms are eager to talk about avoiding pregnancy. She says many have never talked to a doctor about contraception and hold beliefs about birth control that aren't true. For example, one teen told Mollen she heard that birth control pills can lead to obesity in users. "I'm already overweight [so] I don't want to gain more weight," she told Mollen. Another teen said she wondered "if I'm on it for so long would it kill my eggs so I can't have babies?"[13]

It is also important that teens learn about contraceptives because teenage pregnancies pose many risks. Karjane says,

"Pregnancy is much riskier than any form of birth control. . . . And that's [not] just in terms of the medical issues that can develop during pregnancy. When a teen has an unplanned pregnancy, it can disrupt her life, education, or ability to keep a job."[14] The same goes for young men, whose lives may also be disrupted as they are forced to grow up quickly and put the needs of their baby before their own.

"Pregnancy is much riskier than any form of birth control. . . . And that's [not] just in terms of the medical issues that can develop during pregnancy. When a teen has an unplanned pregnancy, it can disrupt her life, education, or ability to keep a job."[14]

—Dr. Nicole W. Karjane, a gynecologist

Sexually Transmitted Infections

Besides pregnancy, teens also need to be concerned about STIs because sex carries the risk of infection. Common sexually transmitted infections include syphilis, gonorrhea, chlamydia, herpes, and human papillomavirus. These ailments may be passed from one person to another through skin contact or contact with bodily fluids such as sperm, vaginal fluid, and saliva. There are STIs that

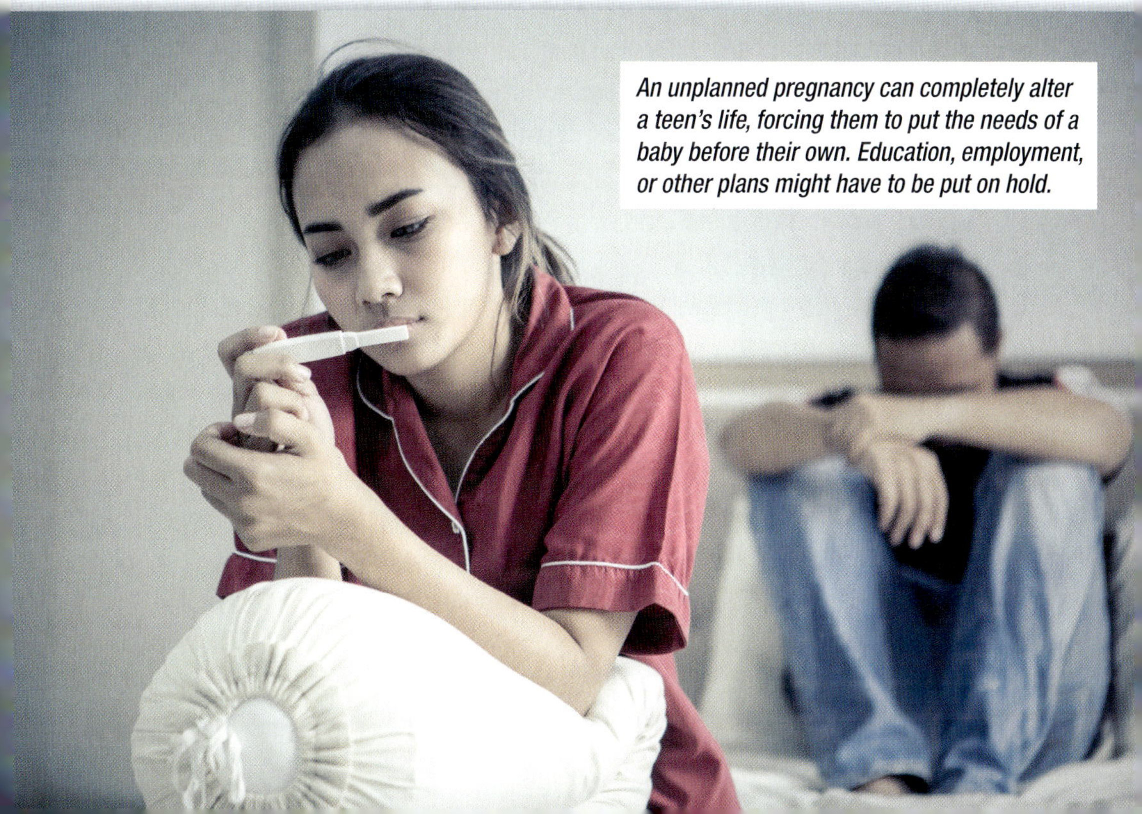

An unplanned pregnancy can completely alter a teen's life, forcing them to put the needs of a baby before their own. Education, employment, or other plans might have to be put on hold.

have no symptoms, making them easy to spread, and others that cause genital warts, rashes, itching, and painful urination. Left untreated, some STIs can lead to serious long-term health consequences such as cancer, organ failure, or the inability to conceive children.

There are ways to guard against STIs. Condoms are one form of protection. They can help prevent the spread of some STIs. However, the odds of acquiring an STI increase with the number of sexual partners. Therefore, having fewer partners is prudent. Where that is an unrealistic expectation, the next best thing, according to the CDC, is to test annually for STIs. Although that agency began recommending such testing in the 1990s, only about 20 percent of sexually active high school students do so, according to the National Institutes of Health, the government agency that keeps health statistics. Antibiotics, which are pills that kill bacteria, are prescribed for some STIs when an infection is detected, and the person must take them for a month even if symptoms have subsided. Teens who know they have a sexually transmitted infection should not have sex with anyone until they have been given the okay by a physician and must inform their recent partners so they can be tested.

As teenagers work their way to adulthood, they will continue to explore new territory, including sexual attraction to other people. Many teens will decide that it is wise to wait to have sex until they are older, have had more dating experience, and are ready to assume the considerable responsibilities that come with being a desirable sexual partner. In making their decisions, they would do well to consider the health consequences that may affect them and the people they care about. In doing so, they will be saving their parenting days for the future—when they are adults and in loving and secure relationships with their partners.

CHAPTER THREE

Avoiding Accidents and Injuries

Caleb is a Wisconsin teen who has been driving for more than two years. Safety is important to him, particularly in light of what happened to his older brother. Caleb's brother was a member of the high school wrestling team. One day, he drove himself to an all-day meet. The event ended in the evening, and the young wrestler drove home in the dark. Exhausted, he fell asleep behind the wheel. "He flipped his car," says Caleb. "[We] found out that he was in the hospital. . . . It definitely made me realize the dangers of driving, that it wasn't all fun and games, like it can change your life in an instant."[15]

Caleb's brother survived; however, accidents and unintentional injuries are the top causes of death among teenagers. Many are avoidable. Therefore, teenagers who are concerned about staying healthy may want to focus on prevention strategies.

> "The advice that I would give to someone who's first starting out driving: make sure any distractions, cell phone, music, radio, whatever it is, make sure that it is off."[16]
>
> —Riley, a Wisconsin teenager

Auto Accidents

In the two years she has been driving, Riley, another Wisconsin teen, has learned the importance of not driving while distracted. When a local hospital asked for volunteers to appear on camera to discuss young driver safety, she agreed to participate. Riley said, "The advice that I would give to someone who's first starting out driving: make sure any distractions, cell phone, music, radio, whatever it is, make sure that it is off."[16]

Distracted driving is a major factor in the cause of automobile accidents, particularly for teen drivers. When more than one thousand teenage drivers were asked in 2024 about their cell phone use while driving, researchers from the six universities conducting the study were shocked. Teens said they spent about 21 percent of their driving time looking at their phones. Even worse, they estimated that a quarter of that time, their eyes left the road for at least two seconds. Two seconds doesn't seem like a long time, but a car traveling at 55 miles per hour (89 kph) will cover 160 feet (49 m) during that brief moment. A lot can go wrong over the span of 160 feet in a car traveling that fast: changes in road conditions, a car swerving between lanes, or a pedestrian stepping into the street in front of an oncoming car.

The study's authors said teens need to learn that multitasking while driving is a recipe for disaster. To avoid the temptation of texting while driving, the researchers suggest teens put their phones in the back seat or place them in Do Not Disturb mode. The latter prevents smartphones from receiving notifications; it can be set up under the phone's settings to go on whenever the phone detects it is in a moving car.

Distracted or not, according to the Virginia-based organization Insurance Institute for Highway Safety, which studies why auto accidents occur, teen drivers are three times more likely to die in automobile accidents than adults over age twenty. The reasons have to do with their not-yet-mature brains, tendency to take risks, and inexperience behind the wheel. Says Canada-based psychotherapist Vikas Keshri, "[Teens] are wired to be bolder and underestimate risk because of their emotional immaturity [and] social pressures."[17]

> "[Teens] are wired to be bolder and underestimate risk because of their emotional immaturity [and] social pressures."[17]
>
> —Vikas Keshri, a Toronto psychotherapist

There are additional steps teens can take to ensure their driving safety. For example, they can limit the amount of time they drive at night, when they are more likely to be sleepy, and transport no more than one passenger in the car. The fewer passengers,

Cell Phones Continue to Be a Distraction for Teen Drivers

Despite efforts to reduce distracted driving among teens, many still use their phones while driving. In a 2025 study, conducted by university public health researchers, seven in ten high school students report using their phones or taking long glances at their phones while driving—often for two seconds or longer. The researchers note that the seconds spent texting, activating a map, or checking social media increase the risk of a crash.

Among participants who reported using their phones while driving, the most common reasons were . . .

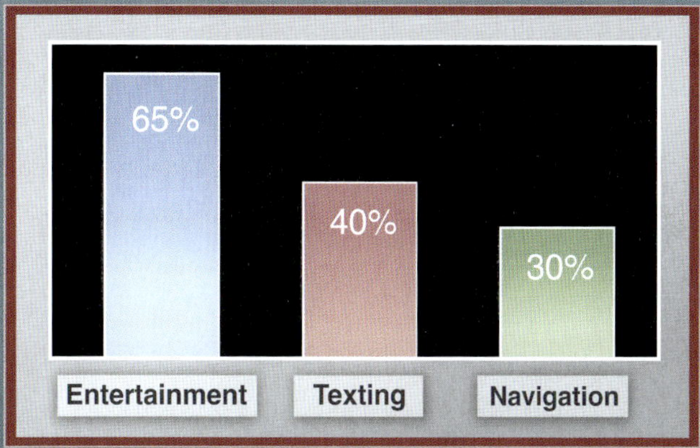

Source: Anna Lamb, "Getting to the Root of Teen Distracted Driving," *The Harvard Gazette*, July 29, 2025. https://news.harvard.edu.

the less likely they will be to show off or be distracted by friends' conversation or antics. Another safety tip is to wear seat belts and insist passengers do the same. Teens should refuse to drink alcoholic beverages and drive or get in the car with someone who is driving while inebriated or under the influence of drugs. Many teens do not follow this advice. A 2025 CDC study found that 19 percent of high school students admit they do not always wear seat belts, and 50 percent text while driving. An earlier CDC study found that 17 percent had been a passenger in a car driven by someone under the influence.

Pedestrian, E-Bike, and E-Scooter Accidents

In addition to avoiding injuries while riding in cars, teens need to be aware of how to safely use e-bikes and e-scooters—and how to avoid danger as pedestrians. The organization Safe Kids Worldwide, based in Washington, DC, says 40 percent of teens surveyed have been hit or nearly hit by cars, motorcycles, or bicycles—as they walked around town. In 13 percent of those incidents, teens admitted they were not paying attention to the traffic moving alongside them. The organization said teens need to be even more careful during evening hours, when darkness makes it harder for drivers to see pedestrians.

To avoid pedestrian injuries, teens should use designated crosswalks and look both ways before stepping off the curb. Wearing headphones and looking at cell phones should be avoided to keep focus on what is happening around them. This is even more important given the rise in popularity of e-bikes and e-scooters.

Don't Ride with Inebriated Friends

The legal drinking age in most states is twenty-one, but sooner or later teenagers may find themselves encountering alcohol or illegal drugs. Power of You(th), a division of the Texas-based organization Mothers Against Drunk Driving that researches underage drinking and driving, suggests that teens plan ahead for that possibility. The organization has developed a pledge that teens can sign as they promise to avoid alcohol and drugs. The pledge states, "Because it's illegal and dangerous, I pledge not to drink alcohol before age 21 or use other drugs. Because I am precious cargo, I pledge never to ride with someone who has been drinking or using drugs. If I find myself in a situation where I feel unsafe or uncomfortable, I pledge to call a trusted adult for a safe ride home."

In the unlikely event that there is no alternative other than getting in the car with an impaired driver, the organization recommends wearing a seat belt, sitting in the back seat, and not engaging the driver in conversation. Once home, it advises telling a parent about the experience so they can decide what steps to take.

Power of You(th), *Power to Take a Stand: Empowering Youth for a Thriving Future*, 2024. https://online.flippingbook.com/view/118502/6.

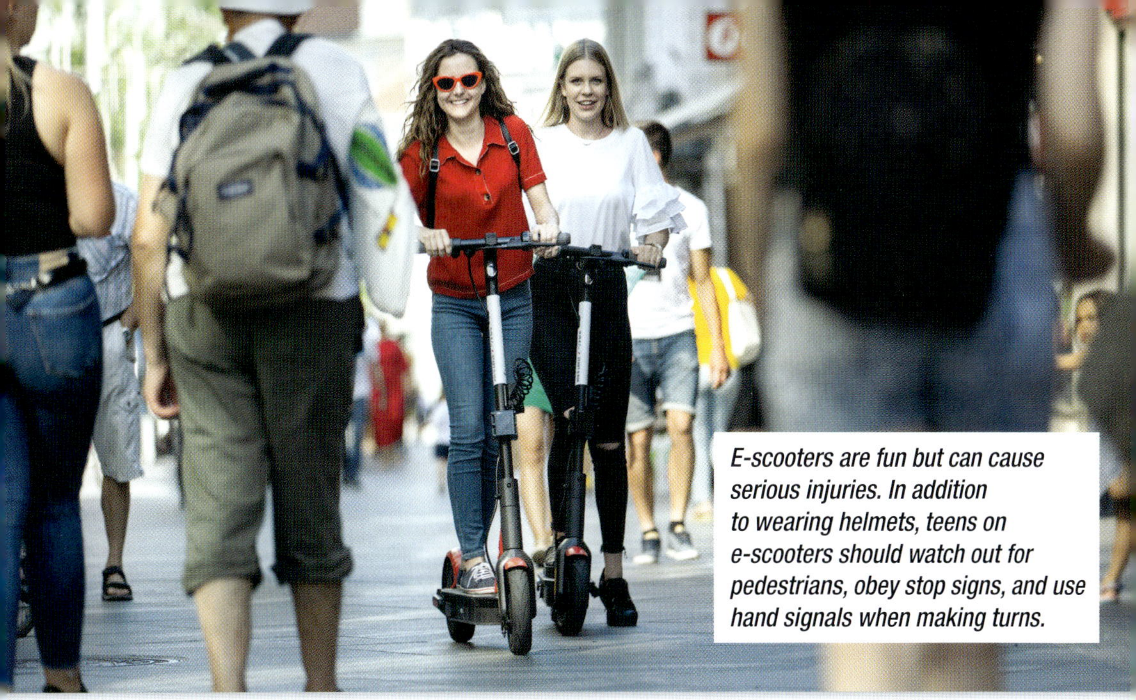

E-scooters are fun but can cause serious injuries. In addition to wearing helmets, teens on e-scooters should watch out for pedestrians, obey stop signs, and use hand signals when making turns.

E-bikes and e-scooters are fun to operate and provide freedom for teenagers who are too young to drive. But they are not toys. E-bikes commonly weigh 40 to 80 pounds (18 to 36 kg), and e-scooters typically weigh 20 to 45 pounds (9 to 20 kg.) E-scooters can reach speeds of 15 to 20 miles per hour (24 to 32 kph), while e-bikes can move even faster, reaching speeds of 20 to 28 mph (32 to 45 kph). Pedestrians struck by a swiftly moving 80-pound e-bike could sustain serious injuries.

Emergency room visits for serious injuries from electric scooters and bikes have been dramatically rising. For example, a 2025 Electric Scooter Accident Report produced by ERideHero, an independent data collection service, found the number of electric scooter injuries rose by 80 percent from 2023 to 2024. The report noted that people ages fifteen to thirty-four accounted for about half of those injuries in 2024. The most common injuries involve the head. According to the same report, there were 20,960 head injuries from electric scooter accidents in 2024. Concussions are not uncommon. A concussion—a bruise to the brain—can occur when the head strikes a hard surface, such as an asphalt street or the steel fender of a car. Concussion symptoms can include nausea, dizziness, blurred vision, confusion, and memory loss.

How Safe Are Teenage Walkers?

Young people started walking as toddlers, but even with years of experiencing walking on their own, many teens don't necessarily pay attention to their surroundings and safety. To find out how safety-conscious teens are while on foot, the Washington, DC–based organization Safe Kids Worldwide stationed observers in school zones to observe more than thirty-four thousand high school and middle school students in undisclosed cities as they left school.

The observers found that many students were leaving school grounds in various states of distraction. One in five high school students and one in eight middle school students were seen crossing the street while distracted. Thirty-nine percent were texting, and 39 percent wore headphones. Twenty-eight percent were on their phones as they stepped into traffic. Meanwhile, 2 percent were playing video games as they walked, with their heads down.

As part of the study, the organization also asked students to guess what age group had the most distracted walking. Nearly 80 percent of the teens choose the "younger than me" category, which was incorrect. In fact, older teens were most at risk.

In addition to wearing helmets, teens need to ride their scooters and bikes responsibly. That means watching out for pedestrians, obeying stop signs (even on sidewalks), and using hand signals when making turns. Also, teens should not ride with passengers, text on their phones, or wear earphones. Teens on electric bikes and scooters also need to be aware of regulations, which vary state by state. For example, teens in New York state must be at least sixteen years old to ride an e-bike and, if under eighteen, must wear a helmet. They are not allowed to go more than 20 miles per hour (32 kph). Similarly, e-scooter riders need to be at least sixteen and are allowed to ride only in designated bike lanes on streets in which the speed limit is 30 miles per hour (48 kph) or less.

Sports Injuries

While driving a car or riding an e-bike on the roadway account for many injuries sustained by teens, others occur on playing fields. According to the CDC, 2.6 million people under age nineteen are injured while playing sports each year.

> "I tore my ACL in the first takedown of the finals match. I could feel it, but I kept wrestling. What else could I do?"[18]
>
> —Hartwell Taylor, a high school wrestler

Many sports-related injuries are avoidable—for example, by not returning to the sport until the injury is fully healed. Wrestler Hartwell Taylor learned that lesson as a high school junior in Kansas City, Missouri. In 2019 Taylor was laser-focused on making his mark at the state championships in his weight class. But when he injured his left knee less than a month before an important competition, he elected to continue wrestling. Despite the knee pain, he won his semifinal match. "That night, I iced my knee, then applied heat the next morning," he says, but the finals proved too much. "I tore my ACL in the first takedown of the finals match. I could feel it, but I kept wrestling. What else could I do?"[18] The ACL—the anterior cruciate ligament—is a crucial connector that stabilizes the bones in the knee.

Taylor required surgery to repair his ACL. After the surgery, he needed to use crutches. Ultimately, he underwent a taxing six-month period of rehabilitation before his ACL was fully healed. He was fortunate to be able to resume wrestling in his senior year, finishing second in his weight class at the state level. Still, it is likely

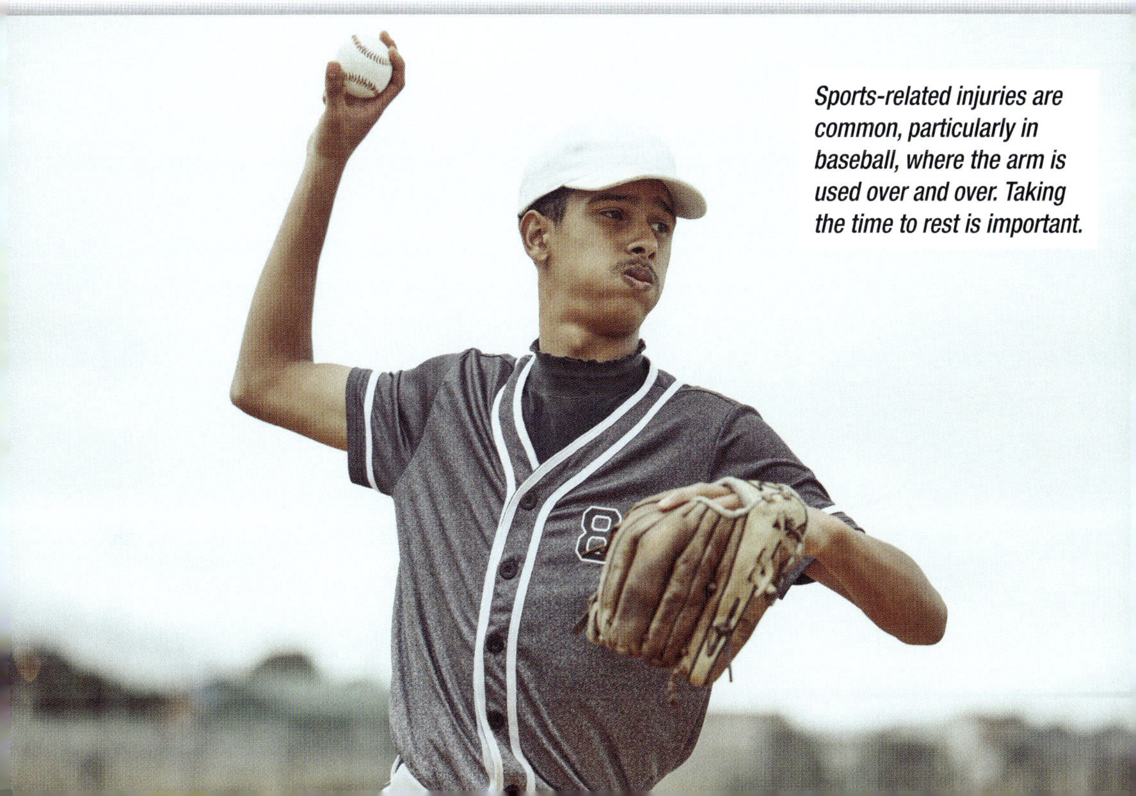

Sports-related injuries are common, particularly in baseball, where the arm is used over and over. Taking the time to rest is important.

that Taylor could have spared himself the surgery and months of recuperation if he had chosen to pay attention to the pain and allow his knee time to recover.

Taylor's story offers another lesson: By practicing the same sport year-round without rest, he had set himself up for injury. Such devotion to a single sport is common among many young competitors in a variety of sports, particularly baseball. "They're starting to throw more, throw different balls faster, and develop those skills at a more elite process at a younger age. As we push these athletes into more specialization faster, they're going to get more hurt frequently,"[19] says Alysia Robichau, a physician at the Houston Methodist Hospital in Texas. She pointed out another problem: As teenagers grow, their growth plates remain pliable—and vulnerable if they are continually stressed. Composed of soft tissue called cartilage, these plates connect bones, enabling them to grow. Robichau says athletes need to take breaks from the physical demands of sports. In other words, a high school athlete with dreams of pitching in the major leagues would do well to give their pitching arm plenty of rest when baseball season ends.

Staying Safe

Safe Kids Worldwide has some additional recommendations for athletes who want to stay safe. For example, before practice starts or games begin, the organization urges young athletes to stretch their arm and leg muscles to loosen them up gradually. And young athletes should wear the appropriate protective gear—with no exceptions. Finally, athletes need to immediately inform their coaches or other adults when they suffer injuries.

Active teens enjoying their independence will inevitably risk accidents and injuries. But taking precautions, thinking ahead, and knowing the rules can lessen the chances of young people suffering injuries and even death. Whether as a pedestrian, automobile driver, e-bike or e-scooter rider, or sports participant, knowing what could go wrong and taking steps to avoid it can lead to continued good health.

CHAPTER FOUR

Teens, Nutrition, and Exercise

As far back as fifth grade, Niche Bryant was a target for school bullies after he gained 80 pounds (36 kg) in little more than a year. Being singled out by bullies made him uncomfortable, but not enough to make any changes. By the time he reached high school, he weighed nearly 300 pounds (136 kg). His parents couldn't help him. He says, "My parents would tell me to take a walk with my grandmother, but I would rather stay home and eat a pack of cookies."[20] What changed for the Brooklyn, New York, high school student was his desire to date. He figured that he would be more likely to find a girlfriend if he lost weight.

> "My parents would tell me to take a walk with my grandmother, but I would rather stay home and eat a pack of cookies."[20]
>
> —Niche Bryant, a Brooklyn high school student

Bryant decided to get outside help to lose weight and soon learned of a nonprofit known as Live Light Live Right. The New York–based organization serves people up to age nineteen who are significantly overweight. It creates individualized care plans and offers counseling to the families of obese teens. Teens learn what foods to eat and how to change their behaviors to be healthier. Fortunately, there was a Live Light Live Right group near Bryant's home, and he followed its advice.

To his surprise, he discovered that eating broccoli became more appealing than the five hamburgers he used to eat in one sitting. He gave up snacking. He also discovered that he enjoyed working out at the gym. Over the next four years, he slimmed down, grew more confident, and engaged in more social activities. His blood pressure, the force with which his blood passes through his arteries, went from high to normal levels, lessening his chances of developing heart disease. (High blood pressure, also known as hypertension, is a common symptom among people who are overweight.) "It's like I had a brick wall on my back, and I was able to break it down,"[21] he says.

After his reboot, Bryant not only dropped his excess weight but also lowered his stress levels, improved his mood, created a habit of exercising, and improved his muscle-to-fat ratio. Teens don't have to be overweight to decide that they want to do something similar by gradually changing their eating and exercise habits. The key to Bryant's success was that he wanted to make the changes. Self-motivated teens can do something similar.

The Health Risks of Obesity

Bryant was not alone in carrying too much weight on his teenage frame. According to the CDC, more than 22 percent of youths ages twelve to nineteen are regarded as obese. And obesity can lead to serious health consequences. In addition to high blood pressure, obese teens face increased risk of developing type 2 diabetes, fatty liver disease, and cancer.

People with type 2 diabetes have too much glucose—or sugar—circulating in their bloodstream because their cells cannot absorb it all. They have become resistant to the effects of insulin, the hormone secreted by the pancreas, the organ whose job is to facilitate glucose's uptake into cells. Left untreated, diabetes may damage a person's arteries, blood vessels, nerves, eyes, liver, and kidneys.

The liver filters toxins from the body while processing nutrients from food. When the liver is surrounded by fat, it must work harder to do its job and can become damaged. Reversible by weight loss, fatty liver disease is a condition suffered by 10 percent of people under age nineteen, according to the Mayo Clinic. "This buildup of fat is commonly caused by obesity, insulin resistance (a cause of diabetes), and diets high in ultra-processed foods [from sodas to chips to sweets] and refined carbohydrates, such

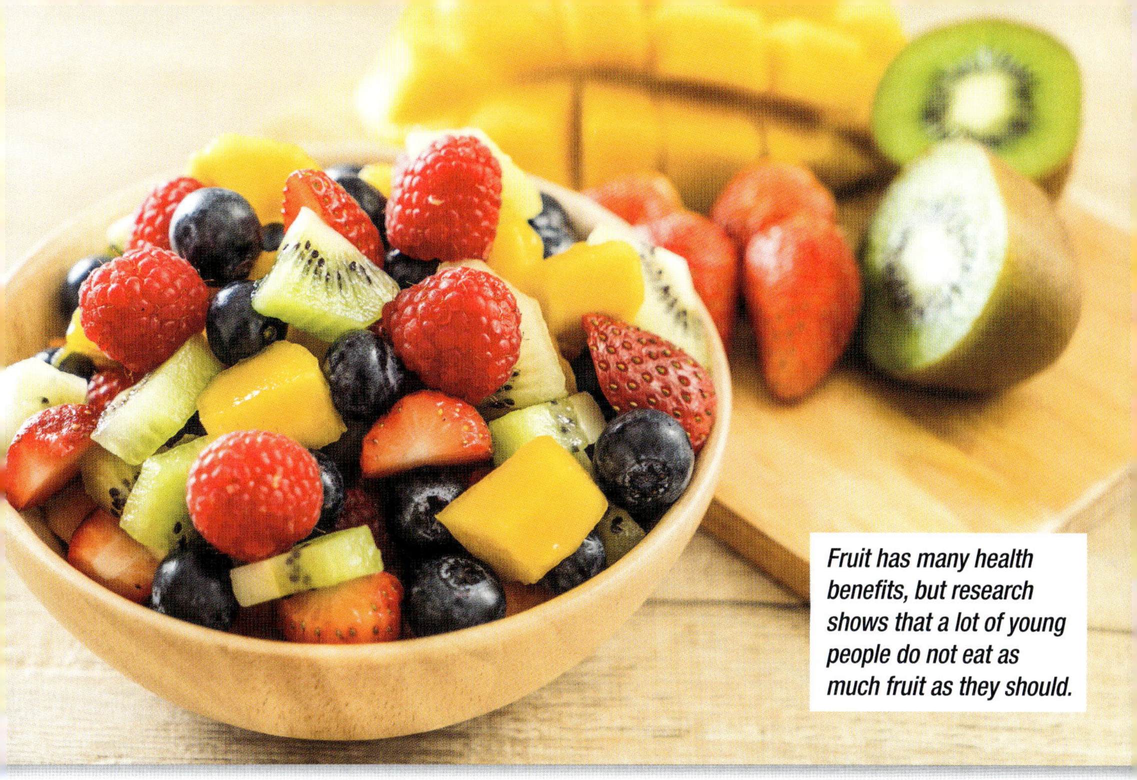

Fruit has many health benefits, but research shows that a lot of young people do not eat as much fruit as they should.

as those seen in the typical American diet,"[22] says Erin Palinski-Wade, a dietitian. Palinski-Wade recommends that people worried about fatty liver disease eat more apples, avocados, grapefruits, and blueberries.

Bryant was also not alone in preferring fast food over vegetables. A 2023 Youth Risk Behavior Survey conducted by Cornell University's Bronfenbrenner Center for Translational Research revealed that only 25 percent of high school students said they ate two servings of vegetables a day. That means that 75 percent of high school students are not getting the recommended amounts of vegetables. Meanwhile, the Cornell survey found that a similar number of students are not eating enough fruit, and nearly three-quarters are skipping breakfast.

Why Nutrition Is Important to Teens

Teens who skip breakfast may have practical reasons for doing so. They may sleep late and have little time to eat before rushing out the door, or they may need to finish a report or project due that day. Many teens don't give much thought to what they eat

Teen Sues over Ultra-Processed Foods

Bryce Martinez, a teenager from Philadelphia, made national news in 2025 when he brought the first lawsuit against multiple manufacturers of ultra-processed foods (UPFs). His lawsuit alleged that consuming some one hundred brands of highly processed foods like Bagel Bites, Sour Patch Kids, Hot Pockets, and Honey Bunches of Oats led him to develop type 2 diabetes and fatty liver disease when he was sixteen.

Unfortunately for Martinez, the lawsuit was dismissed by a judge, who found that it failed to establish a direct connection between the foods Martinez ate and his medical conditions. His lawyers say they remain convinced that the case has merit and might refile it to satisfy the judge's objections. "The scientific evidence demonstrating the addictive nature of these products is compelling," attorney Mike Morgan says. And although the judge dismissed the case, she still recognized the dangers of UPFs, writing, "The court is deeply concerned about the practices used to create and market UPFs, and the deleterious effect UPFs have on children and the American diet."

Quoted in Abraham Gutman, "Lawsuit over Ultra-Processed Foods Is Tossed," *Philadelphia (PA) Inquirer*, August 26, 2025, p. B1.

Quoted in Christian Simmons, "Why a Landmark Ultra-Processed Lawsuit Won't Move Forward," Drugwatch, August 26, 2025. www.drugwatch.com.

anyway, because they have a lot of other things to occupy their minds. They may not be worried about their health at all or may think that health is something they can deal with when they get older. But whether they realize it or not, their poor diet choices may be starting to have an impact.

Teenagers are not adults. Nor are they children. But because they are walking around in growing bodies, their nutritional needs are greater than those of children and adults. To support their growth, they need to consume foods and beverages that facilitate the formation of dense bones that will support their skeletons for a lifetime. Bone formation starts to decline in adulthood, so having a reserve is important.

According to HealthyChildren.org, a division of the American Academy of Pediatrics, health-conscious teens should strive to eat foods that provide their bodies with calcium, vitamins D and

> "I got out of breath sooner than the other kids, and I wasn't as active—or as happy."[23]
>
> —Kelly Worst, a seventeen-year-old softball player

K, and phosphorus. Calcium, a bone-building mineral that also helps maintain teeth, is found in milk, yogurt, broccoli, tofu, chickpeas, kale, canned fish with bones, and other foods. Look for foods whose labels indicate they contain at least 20 percent of the recommended daily allowance of calcium. Vitamin D is found in eggs and in fatty fish such as salmon and sardines. Nuts, seeds, and whole grains are good sources of the mineral phosphorus.

The absorption of calcium by the body can easily be blocked. Sodas and sweetened beverages have been found to block calcium absorption. In addition, drinking alcohol and smoking cigarettes have a negative impact on bone production.

Seventeen-year-old Kelly Worst didn't think a lot about the foods she consumed. Growing up in Cadillac, Michigan, Worst enjoyed being in the school marching band and on the softball team. But unlike the other members of her team, Worst found herself easily exhausted. She realized that was the result of skipping meals and continuously snacking. "I got out of breath sooner than the other kids, and I wasn't as active—or as happy,"[23] she says.

Wanting to do better, Worst joined the support group TOPS—Take Off Pounds Sensibly. The group provided the push she needed to start having regular meals with smaller portions. "I focus on what's going to be better for me," she says. Since she joined the group, she has lost 40 pounds (18 kg). "I'm definitely more comfortable with myself,"[24] she says.

Being on the school softball team meant that she was already getting at least an hour of exercise on most days, as recommended by the US Department of Health and Human Services. But other teens may not be meeting that threshold. They can change that by finding a type of exercise that interests them. Possible choices include aerobic exercise that gets one's heart rate up, strength training that builds muscle, and exercises that strengthen bones. Many can be done at home with little special equipment, such as running, biking, jumping rope, dancing, hiking, and walking.

Performing a series of small movements is also impactful. Walking the dog, taking out the trash, working in the garden, and vacuuming the rugs are examples of little chores that can work toward the daily hour of exercise recommended for teens. When teens decide to limit the amount of time spent sitting, playing video games, and staring at their cell phone screens, they can use that extra time to move more.

Ready to Make Changes

Once teenagers decide to make changes to their diet and exercise, they can boost their chances of success by enlisting help from their families. After all, most food purchases are made by parents, and they don't always choose healthy foods themselves.

Hiking Boosts Mood of Teens in Detention

Something interesting is happening at a six-hundred-student high school in Bath, Maine: Teens who are assigned detention for everything from skipping classes to vaping and talking in class are being offered the opportunity to take a hike instead.

Morse High School happens to be conveniently located near an easy-to-navigate woodland trail. The teacher who leads the hikes is the faculty advisor to the school's outdoor club. She figured hiking would get teens outdoors, where they would experience nature and, with any luck, a change in attitude.

Junior Elsie Nelson-Walling wasn't immediately sold on the idea, thinking that staying in the classroom required less effort. But after going on one of the hikes, she changed her mind. She found it made her feel better. Her unexpected exposure to being outside for a 3-mile (4.8 km) walk has led her to hike even when she doesn't have detention. That's because hiking can boost people's moods and help them relax and de-stress.

Leslie Trundy, the high school guidance counselor behind the hike idea, says, "People seem really different in a good way at the end. . . . They have said things like, 'That was really awesome, thank you.' . . . Even if they're not as vocal about it, I can tell they are in a better place."

Quoted in Kyle Melnick, "A High School in Maine Offers Hikes Instead of Detention. Teachers Are Seeing Results," *Philadelphia (PA) Inquirer*, October 17, 2025. www.inquirer.com.

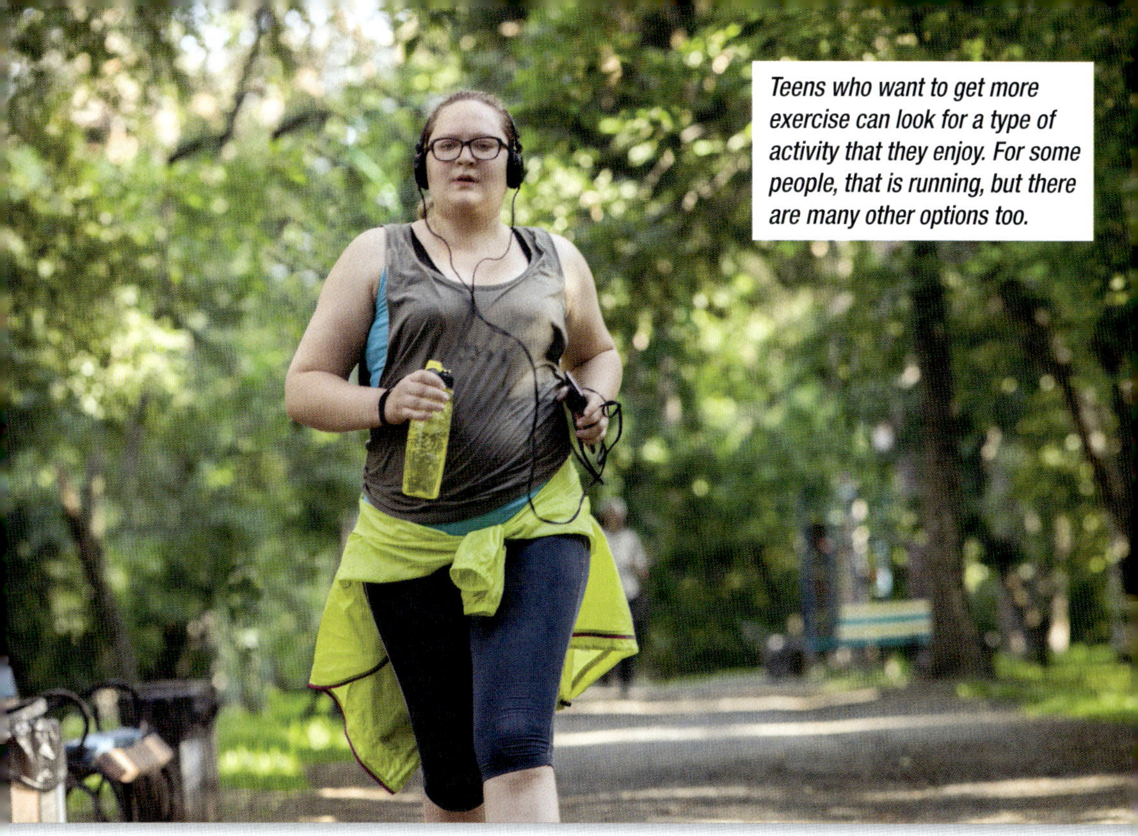

Teens who want to get more exercise can look for a type of activity that they enjoy. For some people, that is running, but there are many other options too.

Teen blogger Ana De Sousa says it is important for teens to talk to their parents about the changes they would like to make and why they want to make them. "If you don't explain why you want to have a healthier lifestyle this could possibly make them worry. Once you have discussed your decision, you can then start working with your parents on helping you, going grocery shopping with them, cooking with them, suggesting going on hikes or runs."[25]

> **"We shouldn't get caught up on the current bogeyman, which is ultra-processed foods. You can find healthy choices even in the ultra-processed category."[26]**
>
> —Kevin Hall, a nutrition scientist and author

Kevin Hall, a nutrition scientist, sums up what it means to eat healthfully with this simple advice: "From what we know about nutritional science, it really does come down to the boring diet advice. You should be eating more fruits, vegetables, and whole grains, and avoiding saturated fat, sugar, salt, and refined carbs. . . . We shouldn't get caught up on the current bogeyman, which is ultra-processed foods. You can find healthy choices even in the ultra-processed category."[26]

Ultra-processed foods are generally defined as not found in nature but created in factories, with additional sugars, salt, and preservatives thrown in to enhance taste and shelf life. Hall concedes that he eats ultra-processed foods, albeit in limited quantities. So, teens don't need to worry about eating them in moderation. Stu Jeck, a high school football coach in Manitou Springs, Colorado, says the same advice holds for fast foods. Jeck, who also teaches health, says, "If you are eating it once a week, maybe a couple times a month, you're on a really good track to living a healthy life."[27]

Teens who get at least the minimum amount of exercise and limit the amount of ultra-processed and fast food they consume will reap big benefits: stronger bones, better concentration, less moodiness, and improved all around health. As a bonus, they will be creating habits that will last a lifetime.

CHAPTER FIVE

Brains Wired for Addiction

Biruk Watling believes she has gotten her life back after swapping out her smartphone for an old-fashioned flip phone that just makes phone calls. Watling is a founder of the Luddite Club at her Brooklyn, New York, high school. Club members choose to reclaim the simple things in life by turning their backs on the alluring influence of social media. Luddite Club members at Watling's school, as well as at other high schools, often gather in parks to talk to each other, sketch nature, or dance. The club's name refers to people who resist technology. The term was first used to refer to nineteenth-century English laborers who feared losing their jobs after their factories were automated. They felt so threatened that they destroyed the new equipment. While calling someone a Luddite is usually a put-down, Watling and her friends happily reclaimed it. Says club member Jameson Butler, "It's sort of a cool kids' club now. It's been great for my high school life socially. No one thinks I am a freak. . . . Many of us have decided we don't want to be in bed, doom-scrolling and rotting our lives away. Youth is being wasted on those of us who are constantly on our phones."[28]

> "Many of us have decided we don't want to be in bed, doom-scrolling and rotting our lives away. Youth is being wasted on those of us who are constantly on our phones."[28]
>
> —Jameson Butler, a high school senior in Brooklyn

Many teens find themselves dealing with addiction—whether it is to social media, smoking, vaping, alcoholic beverages, or illegal drugs. That's not because of young people's personal failings but because of their developing brains. Until their mid-twenties, when their brains reach full maturity, many teens lack impulse control and the ability to consider the long-term effects of their actions. They crave new and even risky experiences that bathe their brains in dopamine, a chemical known as a neurotransmitter that is responsible for creating feelings of happiness. When those pleasurable feelings wear off, as they always do, teens may feel sullen and depressed. These temporary dips may be enough to motivate them to return to their addictions to feel good again.

Social media can make teens feel connected, but it can also make them feel jealous, isolated, and depressed. One of the enticements of having an online life is that it gives people the opportunity to talk about themselves and present an idealized version of their lives. The likes and messages of support they receive can be instant and mood boosting. On the other hand, what they see in posts by others on social media platforms may convince them others are having more fun, own trendier clothes, or have better bodies. And because the cyberworld never shuts down, there can be a fear of missing out if teens step away from their screens. This can lead to lost sleep and a lack of being active in the real world.

Social Media Addiction

Nearly half of teens surveyed in 2024 said they are online constantly, according to a Pew Research Center report on teens, social media, and technology. A decade ago, only 24 percent of teens spent that much time online. Jena Hilliard, a writer who focuses on addiction, compares social media's addictive nature to that of gambling or using cocaine. She says:

> Social media platforms produce the same neural circuitry that is seen in those with a gambling addiction and recreational drug users. . . . Studies have shown that the constant stream of retweets, likes, and shares from these sites cause the brain's reward area to trigger the same kind of chemical reaction seen with drugs like cocaine. In fact, neuroscientists have compared social media interaction to a syringe of dopamine being injected straight into the system.[29]

Many Teens Use Social Media a Lot

More than one-third of teens use social media almost constantly, according to a 2025 Pew Research Center survey. The survey found that 36 percent of teens use at least one of five platforms almost constantly. A larger number use these platforms several times a day. Some experts say that social media sites have been designed to enhance addiction in users.

% of US teens ages 13 to 17 who say they visit or use the following apps or site . . .

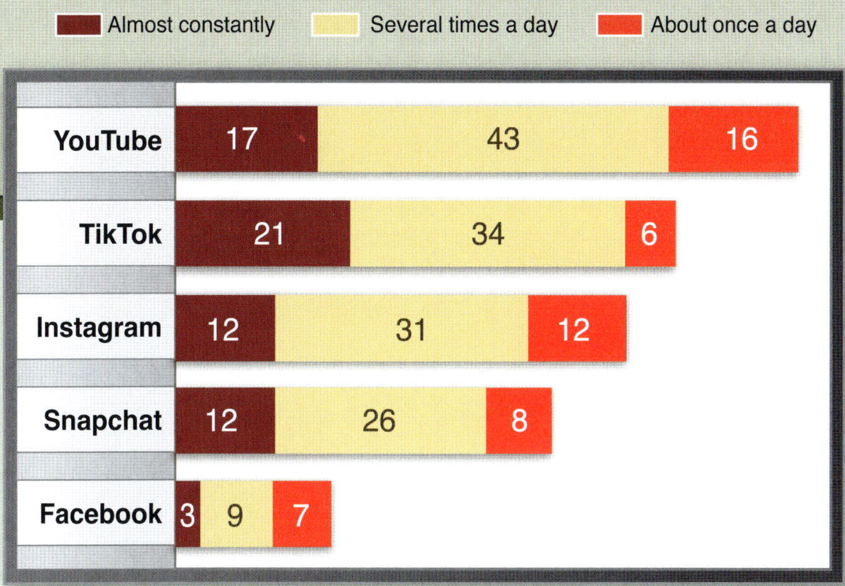

Source: Michelle Faverio and Olivia Sidoti, "Teens, Social Media and AI Chatbots 2025," Pew Research Center, December 9, 2025. www.pewresearch.org.

Social media providers are known to encourage addiction to their sites. The TikTok app, for example, keeps track of the types of content individual users watch and, based on those interests, makes similar videos available. It is therefore easy to keep watching because of the steady stream of videos that pop up. Without realizing it, a TikTok user may spend hours watching video after video. Says Michael Villarreal, a counselor at Tres Vistas Recovery, an addiction treatment center in California, "The biggest red flag is when TikTok starts to interfere with daily responsibilities or relationships. If someone finds themselves skipping work tasks,

Natural Ways to Boost Dopamine

Dopamine is the feel-good chemical produced by our brains that plays a large role in addiction. But there are healthy ways to experience the happy state produced by dopamine without doomscrolling, drinking, smoking, vaping, or engaging in other harmful, addictive behaviors.

Marilyn Spiller, a writer for Stanford Behavior Health, an addiction treatment center in Maine, came up with a list of twenty-seven healthy alternatives that teens can draw on when they need a happiness boost. One suggestion is to take an "awe walk," a stroll in which walkers look for wonders large and small: the flitting of a hummingbird, a pastel sunset, a walk down an unfamiliar street that leads to a surprise park, a visually appealing museum, for example. When teens make a habit of seeking awe, they are more likely to find it and take their focus off their immediate problems.

Other healthy ways to get a dopamine boost Spiller suggests are petting puppies or kittens (or any dogs or cats), licking an ice cream cone, spending time with loved ones, and thinking positive thoughts.

ignoring family or friends, or struggling to keep up with school or chores because they're too wrapped up in endless scrolling, that's a strong sign that their usage has become very unhealthy."[30]

Taking a Break from Tech

Teens may not wish to give up their smartphones as Watling and Butler have done, but they can cut back. For example, they can turn their phones off or put them in another room while they eat, study, or sleep. They can decide how much time they want to spend on Instagram, for example, and set a timer. When the time is up, they can put down their phones and do something else.

"The biggest red flag is when TikTok starts to interfere with daily responsibilities or relationships. If someone finds themselves skipping work tasks, ignoring family or friends, or struggling to keep up with school or chores because they're too wrapped up in endless scrolling, that's a strong sign that their usage has become very unhealthy."[30]

—Michael Villarreal, a counselor at Tres Vistas Recovery

Another way to leave screen time behind is to take walks, perhaps with pet dogs or with family members or friends, leaving their phones at home. Going for a bike ride, mowing the lawn, washing the family car, or playing sports are also ways to enjoy moments with no screens.

Teens who are having problems with specific apps can delete them—as Leonela, a Florida teen, did with Instagram. She says, "I deleted Instagram because it was a trigger for my self-esteem and body image. It took me awhile to realize that whether I like it or not, what I see on my social media feed has an effect on me, mentally and psychologically, and maybe it's not always benefiting me."[31] Leonela now finds that face-to-face interaction with her friends makes her happier than connecting on Instagram.

Older Forms of Addiction

Social media is a relatively new addiction, but there are other, older forms of addiction still causing problems for teens: smoking and vaping, for instance. However, compared to past generations, more teenagers are saying no to the addictions that often afflicted their elders. According to a 2024 study conducted by the University of Michigan's Institute for Social Research, teens today are less likely to use tobacco, drink alcohol, or use illegal

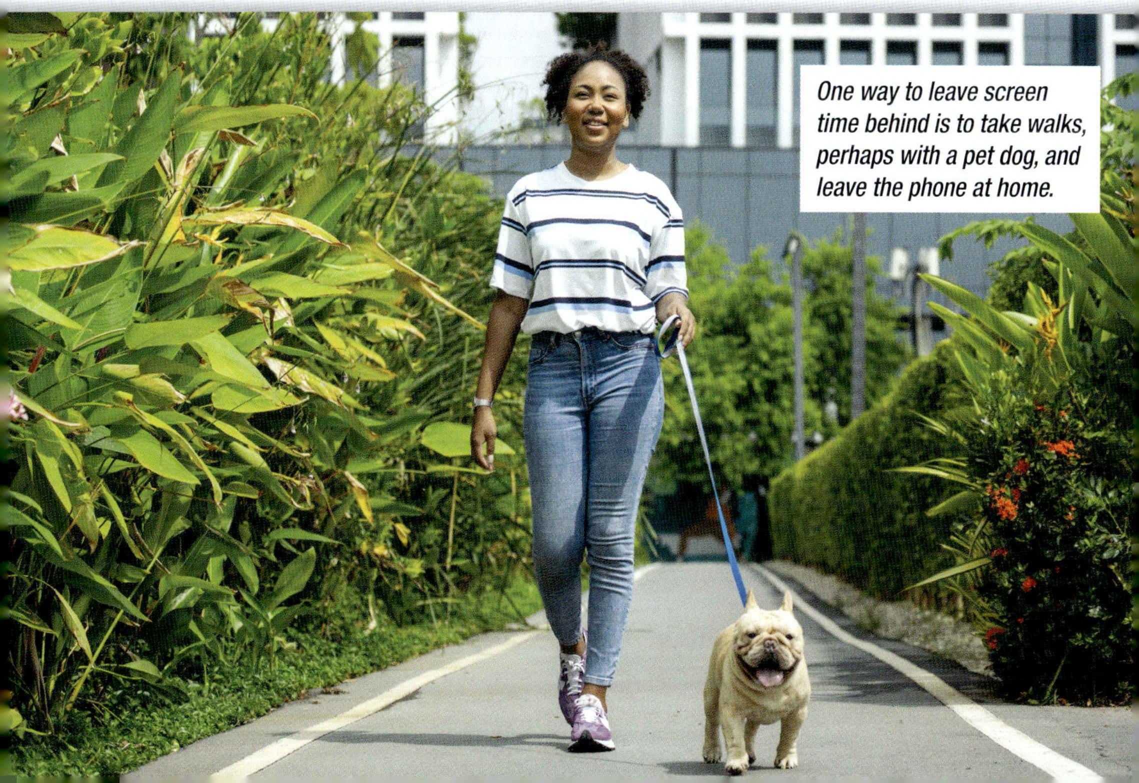

One way to leave screen time behind is to take walks, perhaps with a pet dog, and leave the phone at home.

drugs. In the study, 67 percent of twelfth graders said they were avoiding drugs, compared to 53 percent who said so in 2017, the first year that question was asked. Forty-two percent of high school seniors said they had consumed alcohol in the past year, compared to 75 percent who said so in 2017.

The study suggests that today's teens may know more about the health impacts of substance abuse. Also, teens may fear seeing their out-of-control behavior prompted by alcohol or drug use show up on social media. As for cigarette smoking, the increased cost of cigarettes may have placed them out of the reach of young people. According to the California-based World Population Review, which studies international economics, in 2025 the average cost of a pack of cigarettes in the United States was $10. Therefore, a pack-a-day habit could cost $70 a week—a sum a typical teen would find difficult to pay.

One Teenage Alcoholic's Story

Teens who have experienced drinking problems sometimes are willing to share their stories anonymously in the hope of preventing other teens from following their path or just to let them know that they are not alone. Such was the case for one young woman who shared how quickly she became addicted to alcohol. She said that when she drank with friends, she realized she constantly thought about getting intoxicated. Drinking made her feel more at ease with people.

In less than two years, she went from drinking one cocktail at night to an entire bottle of liquor. She stopped getting straight As, disappointed her parents, was threatened with expulsion, and couldn't remember things that had happened to her.

She decided to quit drinking days before her seventeenth birthday. Attending Alcoholics Anonymous (AA) was a big help. AA is a worldwide peer support group that promotes a 12-step recovery plan. She says, "Just because I knew I was an alcoholic and would later want to stop drinking, doesn't mean I could just stop. It wasn't that simple. But AA being there throughout, welcoming me when I felt like nothing, and slowly helping me build up whatever it was that allowed me to stop, was invaluable."

Quoted in Our Happy Notes, "Teenage Alcoholic's Sober Story," January 8, 2023. https://ourhappynotes.com.

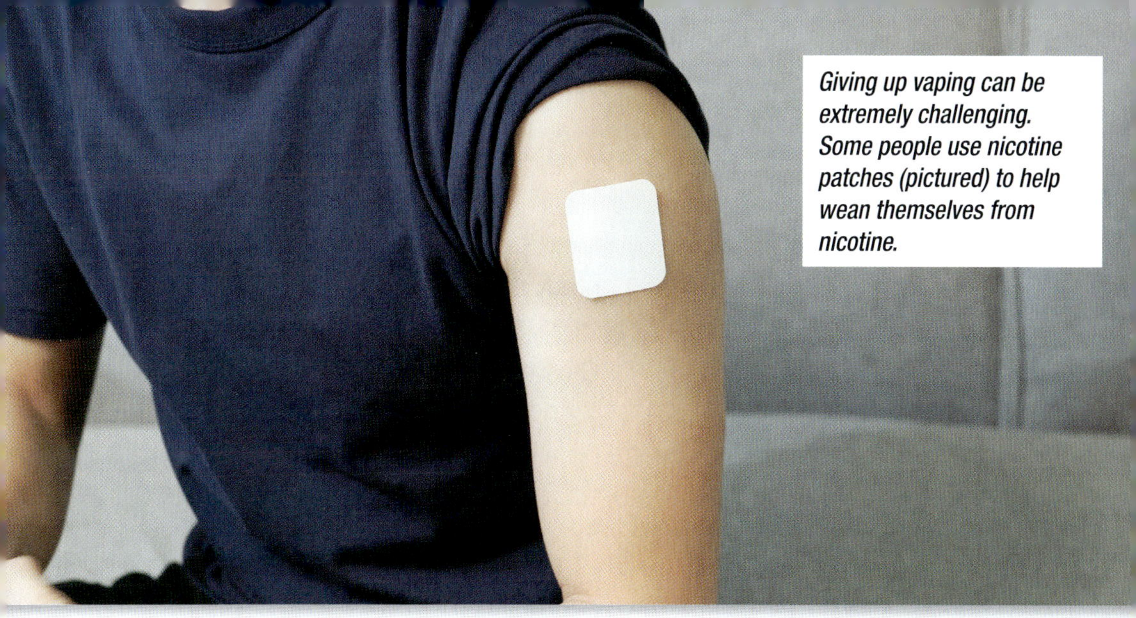

Giving up vaping can be extremely challenging. Some people use nicotine patches (pictured) to help wean themselves from nicotine.

Although the number of teens experimenting with those substances is on the decline, there are still millions of teens using them. "The goal is to impress upon youth that far and away the healthiest choice is not to put these substances in your body," says Aaron Weiner, a psychologist from Lake Forest, Illinois. "The longer we can get kids to go without using substances regularly, the better their chances of having an optimal life trajectory."[32]

Some teens, such as eighteen-year-old Justice Monro, began vaping to fit in with their classmates. Monro, from Sandpoint, Idaho, often felt like an outsider at school but discovered that vaping was a way to find acceptance by her classmates. She says:

> The first time I vaped was on one of the first days of middle school in seventh grade. I went in the girls' bathroom and there was a big group of popular girls. . . . They asked me if I wanted to try their vape that they had. The first time I tried it, I felt like I was gonna throw up. My chest got super tight. And I was trying to play it off like nothing was happening. They saw that I wasn't a snitch, that I wasn't gonna tell on them, so they asked me to hang out with them more. Previously, I didn't really fit in at all, and so just like having that feeling like someone wanted to be my friend just meant everything to me.[33]

> "I went in the girls' bathroom and there was a big group of popular girls. . . . They asked me if I wanted to try their vape that they had. The first time I tried it, I felt like I was gonna throw up. My chest got super tight. And I was trying to play it off like nothing was happening."[33]
>
> —Justice Monro, an Idaho teen

When she took her first puff, Monro had no idea that her body would develop a tolerance for nicotine, meaning to feel good she would need increasing amounts of the chemical that makes tobacco so addictive. She had no idea that nicotine could cause severe health issues, among them high blood pressure, rapid heartbeat, coughing, and gum damage. In addition, she didn't know that she would feel ill as she went through the withdrawal phase after deciding to quit.

Quitting Can Be a Challenge

Jaylon Robinson started vaping in seventh grade and decided to give up the habit three years later. Giving up vaping caused him to suffer headaches and experience mood shifts. He also had trouble breathing. He had to take time off from school and use nicotine patches prescribed by his physician to gradually wean himself from the drug. Robinson had to apply a nicotine patch to his skin that would send a small but constant amount of nicotine to his system. The patches supply enough nicotine to prevent the wearer from missing the larger hit of nicotine to which they were accustomed. Eventually, users of the patch find themselves less and less dependent on nicotine. Still, quitting his vaping habit was a challenge. He says, "I'm really proud of myself, and there's been a few people that have seen the things that I've done, and one of my friends said that he quit because of it. And, you know, that was cool."[34]

Under the right circumstances, anyone can become addicted, and teens are more likely to face addiction because of their developing brains. Whether the addiction is to screens, nicotine, alcohol, or illegal drugs, help is available for teens who cannot address their issues on their own. The first step is for teens to admit they have a problem and to tell their parents or another trusted adult who can provide them with the resources they need to put their addictions behind them.

CHAPTER SIX

Tired Teens

Teachers don't like it when teens fall asleep in class. But at Mansfield Senior High School in Mansfield, Ohio, sleep is on the curriculum. Actually, it is a class students can take to help them learn how to sleep better at home. Nathan Baker took the class and as a result changed his bedtime routine. Baker tries to fall asleep around 10:00 p.m. But he begins settling down as early as 7:00 or 8:00 p.m. That's when he stops paying attention to his phone and his appetite. He stops eating because he knows that eating too close to bedtime can have an adverse effect on his sleep.

Baker makes his room nice and dark by shutting his curtains because he knows that light can trick his body into believing it is daytime. He listens to music that is soothing, such as jazz or R&B, because those choices relax him. He says, "I feel a lot better. I'm coming to school with a smile on my face. Life is so much more simple."[35]

Baker gets seven hours of sleep each night, which is more than he had been getting before taking the class, when his bedtime routine included watching videos in bed on his phone. Teenagers need eight to ten hours of sleep each night, a threshold that most of them don't come close to meeting, according to the Bronfenbrenner Center for Translational Research. In fact, the sleep deprivation gets worse as teens age, with 31 percent of ninth graders getting eight hours of sleep, while only 18 percent of high school seniors do, according to Heather Turgeon and Julie Wright, coauthors of *Generation Sleepless*. Teens who get less sleep than that risk having poorer grades, moodiness, distractibility, and weight gain, and they are more likely to engage in substance abuse and risky behaviors, miss class, and be late for school, according to Lisa L. Lewis, author of the 2022 book *The Sleep-Deprived Teen*.

Having a persistent sleep deficit is a problem, according to Turgeon and Wright, who are psychotherapists and sleep therapists. They say, "Our teenagers are in the midst of the worst case of [sleep] deprivation experienced by any population in history."[36] And lessened rest can lead to having anxious thoughts, experiencing greater stress, and feeling down.

The Need for Sleep

Sleep is particularly important for teenagers, whose bodies are growing even as their brains are forming new memories and mastering new skills. During sleep their bodies repair damaged muscles, eliminate toxins, and strengthen their immune systems so they don't get sick as often. Sleep also helps regulate metabolism, or how efficiently their bodies process the food they eat. Having sufficient sleep means fewer cravings for unhealthy foods and less weight gain. And all of that happens automatically, without them doing anything other than spending enough time asleep.

As they sleep, teens cycle through five stages in a ninety-minute period, according to Turgeon and Wright, and each stage has a purpose. For example, in the first stage (a drowsy state when sleep is the lightest), memories are either burnished or jettisoned to make

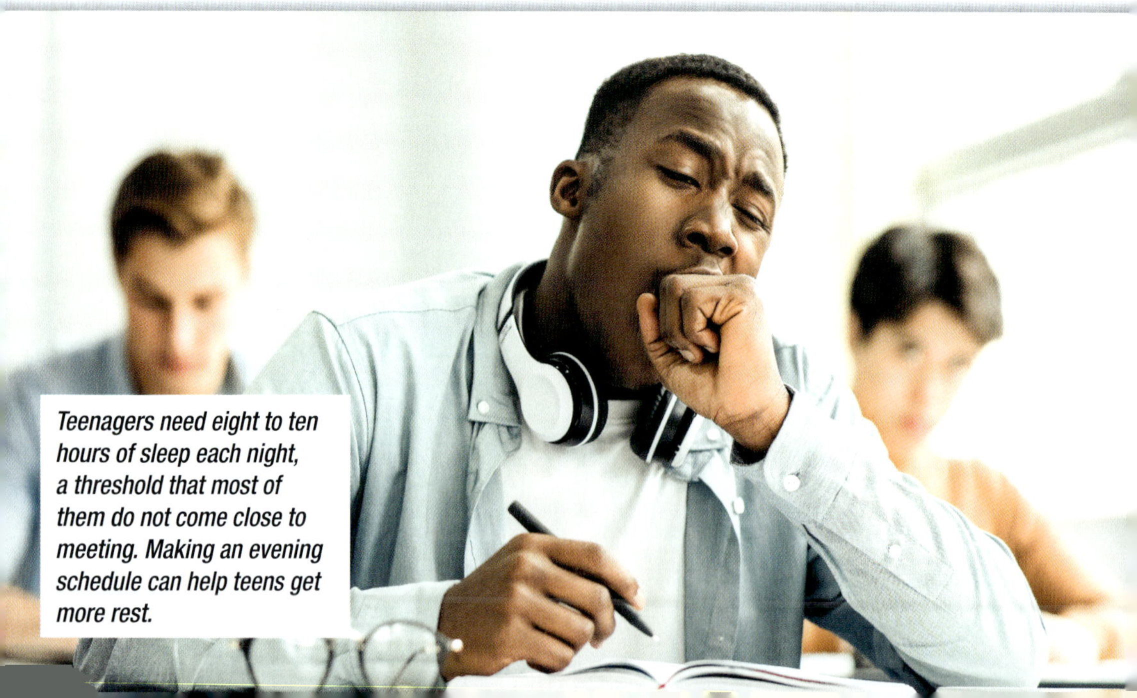

Teenagers need eight to ten hours of sleep each night, a threshold that most of them do not come close to meeting. Making an evening schedule can help teens get more rest.

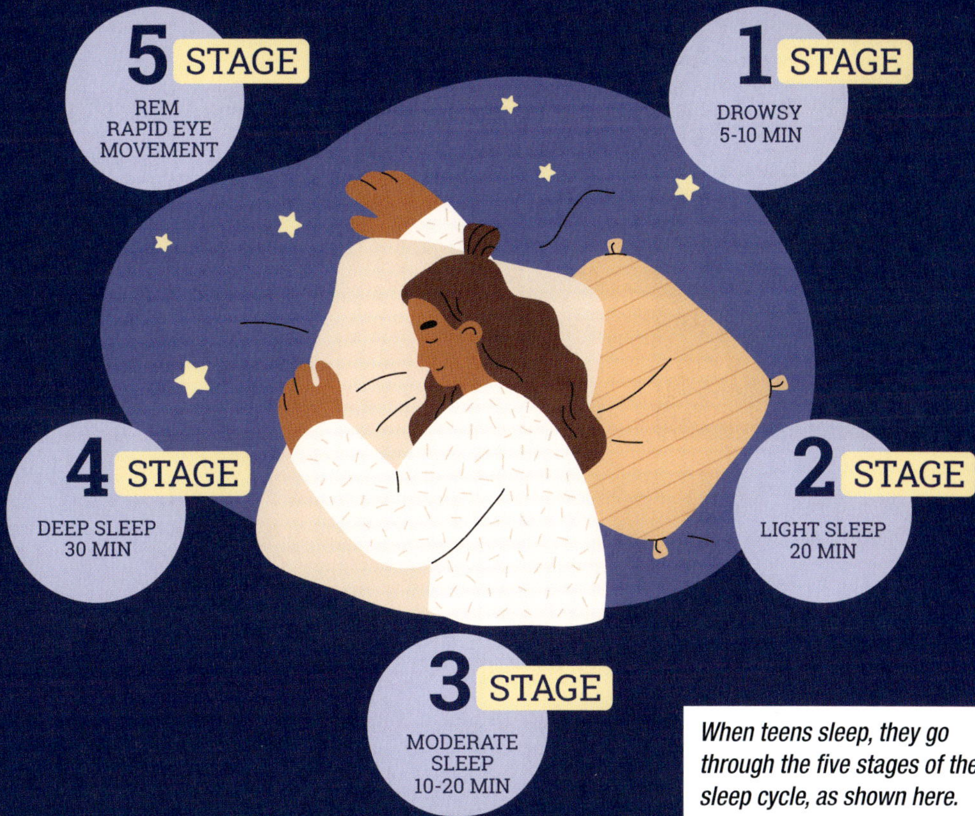
5 STAGE
REM
RAPID EYE
MOVEMENT
1 STAGE
DROWSY
5-10 MIN
4 STAGE
DEEP SLEEP
30 MIN
2 STAGE
LIGHT SLEEP
20 MIN
3 STAGE
MODERATE
SLEEP
10-20 MIN

When teens sleep, they go through the five stages of the sleep cycle, as shown here.

way for new ones. And in deep sleep, the fourth stage, teens release the hormones that aid their growth. Meanwhile, in the last stage, rapid eye movement (REM) sleep, dreaming occurs. Turgeon and Wright say this stage plays a role in the ability of teens to learn new material and think creatively.

What Gets in the Way of Sleep

While teenagers require a lot of sleep, there are factors working against them getting it. Among them are early school start times, busy schedules worsened by academic pressures to earn high grades, and teens' natural rhythms that predispose them to want to sleep in during the morning and stay up late at night.

As a high school freshman, Issac Olson of Rosemount, Minnesota, struggled to adjust to his school's 7:29 a.m. start time. After all, his middle school classes had started at 8:00 a.m. He says, "I strive to get 8–9 hours of sleep every night, but my early start times make this a challenge. During the week, I usually get around seven and a half hours of sleep. Every Friday, I feel so tired from the week of getting up early that I usually go to bed at the same time I would on a school night. However, on the weekends, I get around two hours more sleep every night than I do during the week."[37]

> **"I recognize that it is difficult to change school start times, but schools across the nation have done it, and seen benefits. I think that delaying school start times should be a high priority, because it will redefine the educational experience for hundreds of students and teachers."[38]**
>
> —Issac Olson, a high school student

Olson would like his school district to delay his school's start time until 8:00 or 8:30 a.m., which would be a better fit for teenagers' sleep cycles. Olson wishes Minnesota would follow California and Florida, two states that have mandated later school start times for teenagers. He says:

> I recognize that it is difficult to change school start times, but schools across the nation have done it, and seen benefits. I think that delaying school start times should be a high priority, because it will redefine the educational experience for hundreds of students and teachers. Even if I still get 7 and a half hours of sleep each night, I know that with later start times, this sleep will be more aligned with my natural sleep patterns.[38]

Most teens would feel powerless to do anything about their schools' start times. But Matt was not one of those young people. In 2021 the fifteen-year-old was a student representative at Newton High School in Newton, Massachusetts, when he decided to research the issue after averaging six hours of sleep each night. Matt decided to survey his fellow students about their sleep habits and presented the results to his principal. Matt was able to show him that 73 percent of the students were not getting enough sleep. Through Matt's efforts, the school start time moved to 9:00 a.m., letting the students sleep later each morning and arrive ready to learn.

Small Changes Can Make a Difference

Matt's story is inspirational, but even teens who must report for their schools' early start times can begin to make some small changes to their routines. Turgeon and Wright have suggested five habits that can be practiced by teens who want to get better-quality sleep.

The first habit is maintaining a consistent sleep and wake schedule, even on weekends. Turgeon and Wright acknowledge that maintaining a consistent sleep schedule is challenging for teens and some nights will require exceptions; but overall, it is both doable and worthwhile. To get started, teens need to calculate how much sleep they need and work backward from when they need to get up. Once they determine the ideal time to be in

To Caffeinate or Not to Caffeinate?

Some teens consume caffeine every day in the form of soda, coffee, tea, or energy drinks. Caffeine is a stimulant, and many people rely on it to start their day, particularly if they have not slept well. Since about 2011 the American Academy of Pediatrics, a professional organization for pediatricians, has been recommending that young people under eighteen consume less than 100 milligrams of caffeine a day—the equivalent of about two cups of tea, an 8-ounce (227 g) cup of coffee, two cans of cola, or two energy drinks.

Caffeine can help teens focus and provide them with a pick-me-up. But it can also play a role—both positive and negative—in sleep. Too much caffeine in a teen's body can prevent them from being sleepy as much as five to seven hours after consumption. So, teens need to stop drinking caffeinated beverages by early afternoon, experts say.

But there is something called a caffeine nap that might be worth trying. To take one, teens need to drink one cup of coffee and then nap for twenty minutes. Lisa L. Lewis, author of *The Sleep-Deprived Teen*, says, "If done properly, including at the right time of day (not too close to bedtime), it's considered more effective than either strategy alone. You might get some restoration from the brief nap, followed by a boost of alertness when the caffeine kicks in."

Lisa L. Lewis, *The Sleep-Deprived Teen: Why Our Teenagers Are So Tired, and How Parents and Schools Can Help Them Thrive.* Mango, 2022, p. 168.

bed, they may try slowly adapting to their new bedtime routine by going to bed ten minutes earlier each night until they work their way back to that optimal time.

The second habit is to develop familiar routines that ease them into wakefulness or sleepiness. The wind-down should begin about an hour before bedtime. It's the time to lower the lights, relax, and put cell phones away. Such routines are important for transitioning from wakefulness to sleep. Says Alex Dimitriu, a California physician specializing in sleep disorders, "The human brain can't go from 100 miles an hour to zero in 20 minutes."[39]

About fifteen to thirty minutes after the wind-down, teens can begin their bedtime routine. The routine may involve taking a shower, donning pajamas, brushing their teeth, and reading for pleasure. If the routine is relaxing and done in low light, it will be effective at telling a teen's body that the time for sleep is approaching.

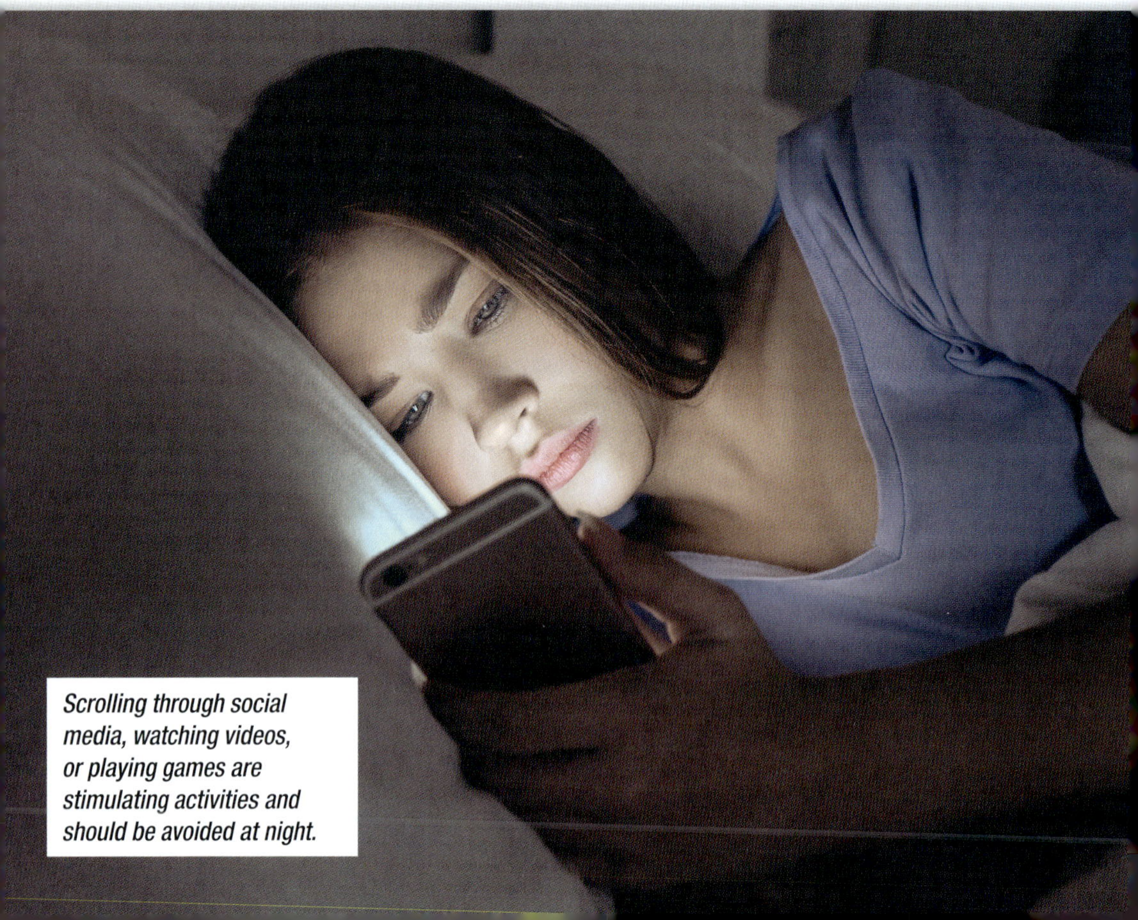

Scrolling through social media, watching videos, or playing games are stimulating activities and should be avoided at night.

Dog Sleeping

According to the American Academy of Sleep Medicine, an organization made up of eleven thousand sleep centers and sleep specialists, 53 percent of Generation Z—the generation most teenagers belong to—sleep with a pet. While some might suppose that such an arrangement would lead to poorer sleep, a few studies have found the opposite to be true.

Among them is a 2021 study conducted by researchers at Concordia University Pediatric Public Health Psychology Lab in Canada. Using data from its Healthy Heart Project, which included information gleaned from nine- to eighteen-year-olds, the study found that "sleeping with your pet does not appear to be disruptive," lead study author Hillary Rowe says. "Indeed, we found that children who slept with their pets most often reported higher perceived sleep quality, especially among adolescents."

Rowe believes that people who sleep beside their dogs or cats find it comforting. As long as they continue to report restful sleep, there is no reason to make the family pet sleep in its own bed.

Quoted in Patrick Lejtenyi, "Kids Who Sleep with Their Pet Still Get a Good Night's Rest, According to Concordia Research," Concordia University, June 2, 2021. www.concordia.ca.

Turgeon and Wright's third habit is eliminating anything that sabotages sleep. For example, stimulating activities keep teens awake. Turgeon and Wright write:

> If a teen climbs into bed and scrolls through social media, plays a game, watches YouTube, or video chats with a friend, she . . . [is] in a state of activation, wondering, worrying, and checking something in the external world. This will make it harder to fall asleep. It can also cause night wakings, because if she falls asleep this way . . . during the night she may instinctively reach to check the phone or think about the game, video or conversation. When externally focused sleep associations are in place, our sleep is delayed, choppy, short, and inadequate, and our delicate sleep bubble has popped.[40]

"It may sound odd to say that kids in high school have to learn the skills to sleep. But you'd be shocked how many just don't know how to sleep."[42]

—Tony Davis, a high school health teacher

The fourth step is to eliminate light in the bedroom—even the light from a digital alarm clock. If a teen's bedroom isn't dark, sleep will be disrupted. So that means pulling down shades and creating a cool environment with a lower room temperature, from 60 to 68 degrees Fahrenheit (15.6°C to 20°C). "Sounds chilly to some, but a cooler room helps you fall asleep faster, because as your body's core temperature lowers, this sends signals to the brain that it's time to sleep,"[41] Turgeon and Wright say.

The fifth step is practicing a sleep-friendly daytime that helps the body clearly tell whether it is time to be awake or asleep. Teens who go outside or otherwise expose themselves to bright light ten minutes or so after waking signal to their bodies that it's time to be awake. Fitting in some daily exercise helps create a more tired feeling later in the day. Turgeon and Wright say moderate exercise performed at least several hours before bedtime reduces stress, lifts mood, and enhances the deep sleep that helps teens grow.

A Magic Pill

Turgeon and Wright compare sleep to a magic pill available to everyone, totally free and completely natural. Virtually everyone can take some steps to improve their sleep each night. The need to do so is obvious. "It may sound odd to say that kids in high school have to learn the skills to sleep. But you'd be shocked how many just don't know how to sleep,"[42] says Tony Davis, the health teacher who taught the class Nathan Baker took that helped him change his sleep habits.

Once teens recognize why sleep is important and which everyday activities get in the way of having good sleep, they can begin trying to get eight or more hours of sleep each night. When they do, they might be rewarded by having more energy, improved moods, and better grades. They may also gain the ability to avoid accidents, make better decisions, get sick less, and experience fewer episodes of anxiety, stress, and depression.

SOURCE NOTES

Introduction: Choosing Wellness

1. Julia Weissman, "Spotting the Fakes: How Teens Are Navigating Health Misinformation," Peer Health Exchange, October 28, 2024. www.peerhealthexchange.org.
2. Weissman, "Spotting the Fakes."
3. National Institute of Diabetes and Digestive and Kidney Diseases, "Take Charge of Your Health: A Guide for Teenagers," 2023. www.niddk.nih.gov.

Chapter One: Teens and the Challenges of Mental Health

4. Quoted in Katie Lott, "Cady's Story: How One Teen Fought Anxiety," Children's Wisconsin, April 22, 2019. https://childrenswi.org.
5. Quoted in Lott, "Cady's Story."
6. Quoted in Hyoung Chang, "Read Their Stories. Hear Their Words," *Denver Post*. https://youthsuicide.denverpost.com.
7. Quoted in Elisha R. Galaif et al., "Suicidality, Depression, and Alcohol Use Among Adolescents: A Review of Empirical Findings," National Library of Medicine, July 12, 2011. https://pmc.ncbi.nlm.nih.gov.
8. Quoted in Chang, "Read Their Stories."
9. Quoted in Justin W. Patchin, "Teens Talk: What Works to Stop Cyberbullying," Cyberbullying Research Center, 2025. https://cyberbullying.org.
10. Quoted in Patchin, "Teens Talk."

Chapter Two: Teens and Sex

11. Quoted in Empower ARC, "Real Life Stories." www.empowerarc.org.
12. Quoted in Empower ARC, "Real Life Stories."
13. Quoted in Cynthia Mollen, "Teens Want Accurate Information About Birth Control—the Emergency Department Can Deliver It," Children's Hospital of Philadelphia Poly Lab, June 12, 2024. https://policylab.chop.edu.
14. Nicole W. Karjane, "What I Wish All Teens Knew About Long-Acting Birth Control," Every Stage Health, 2023. www.acog.org.

Chapter Three: Avoiding Accidents and Injuries

15. Quoted in Children's Wisconsin, *Teen Driving Safety: Lessons Learned*, YouTube, December 23, 2021. www.youtube.com/watch?v=skvXHEcBvXw.
16. Quoted in Children's Wisconsin, *Teen Driving Safety*.

17. Quoted in Kris Ann Valdez, "Why Summer Is the Most Dangerous for Teen Drivers—and What Parents Can Do," MSN, May 8, 2025. www.msn.com.
18. Quoted in Children's Mercy Hospital, "Torn ACL: Hartwell's Story," 2025. www.childrensmercy.org.
19. Quoted in Spencer Plato, "Tommy John Surgeries Are Increasing in Teen Athletes Playing Baseball," Houston Public Media, June 10, 2024. www.houstonpublicmedia.org.

Chapter Four: Teens, Nutrition, and Exercise

20. Quoted in Julie Mazziotta and Stephanie Emma Pfeffer, "Weight Loss for Teens Is Controversial: 4 Share How—and Why—They Took Charge of Their Health," *People*, August 29, 2019. https://people.com.
21. Quoted in Mazziotta and Pfeffer, "Weight Loss for Teens Is Controversial."
22. Quoted in Kristina Mastrocola, "Not All Sugar Is Created Equal: 4 Fruits That Heal a Fatty Liver," NewsBreak, August 29, 2025. www.newsbreak.com.
23. Quoted in Mazziotta and Pfeffer, "Weight Loss for Teens Is Controversial."
24. Quoted in Mazziotta and Pfeffer, ""Weight Loss for Teens Is Controversial."
25. Ana De Sousa, "How to Actually Start Your Health Journey as a Teenager," *Meghan's Teen Life* (blog), March 6, 2021. https://meghansteen.health.blog.
26. Quoted in Anahad O'Connor, "NIH Researcher Offers Ideas on Food Intelligence," *Philadelphia (PA) Inquirer*, October 19, 2025, p. G3.
27. Quoted in Jarrin Hall, "Students Choose Fast Food for Convenience Despite the Health Risks," *The Prospector*, February 5, 2025. https://mshsprospector.org.

Chapter Five: Brains Wired for Addiction

28. Quoted in Alex Vadukul, "Now in College, Luddite Teens Still Don't Want Your Likes," *Hawaii Tribune Herald* (Hilo, HI), February 3, 2025. www.hawaiitribune-herald.com.
29. Jena Hilliard, "Social Media Addiction," Addiction Center, July 28, 2025. www.addictioncenter.com.
30. Quoted in Ashley Broadwater, "The 1 Sign You're Addicted to TikTok," HuffPost, January 19, 2025. www.huffpost.com.
31. Quoted in Boys & Girls Clubs of America, "Supporting Digital Well-Being: 12 Ways to Help Teens Unplug from Technology," 2025. www.bgca.org.

32. Quoted in Zara Abrams, "More Teens than Ever Are Overdosing. Psychologists Are Learning New Approaches to Combat Youth Substance Misuse," *Monitor on Psychology*, March 2024. www.apa.org.
33. Quoted in *Nic Sick: The Dangers of Youth Vaping*, PBS, 2023. www.pbs.org.
34. Quoted in Marie Edinger, "Florida Teen Quits Vaping After Long Journey to Battle Addiction," Fox 35, February 3, 2024. www.fox35orlando.com.

Chapter Six: Tired Teens

35. Quoted in Jacelyn Gecker, "Sleep Training Is No Longer Just for Babies. Some Schools Are Teaching Kids How to Sleep," KSAT-TV, April 16, 2025. www.ksat.com.
36. Heather Turgeon and Julie Wright, *Generation Sleepless*. Tarcher, 2022, p. 3.
37. Issac Olson, "Personal Stories," Minnesota Sleep Society, 2020. www.minnesotasleepsociety.org.
38. Olson, "Personal Stories."
39. Quoted in Chantelle Lee, "Why You Still Have Stress Dreams About School," *Time*, August 29, 2025. https://time.com.
40. Turgeon and Wright, *Generation Sleepless*, p. 166.
41. Turgeon and Wright, *Generation Sleepless*, p. 175.
42. Quoted in Gecker, "Sleep Training Is No Longer Just for Babies."

FOR FURTHER RESEARCH

Books

Leah Aguirre and Geraldine O'Sullivan, *The Girl's Guide to Relationships, Sexuality, and Consent: Tools to Help Teens Stay Safe, Empowered, and Confident*. Instant Help, 2022.

David A. Clark, *The Anxious Thoughts Workbook for Teens*. Instant Help, 2022.

Tina Land-Caulk, *Eat Well and Feel Great: The Teenager's Guide to Nutrition and Health*. Green Tree, 2023.

Lisa L. Lewis, *The Sleep-Deprived Teen: Why Our Teenagers Are So Tired, and How Parents and Schools Can Help Them Thrive*. Mango, 2022.

Elisa Nebolsine, *Your Amazing Teen Brain: CBT & Neuroscience Skills to Stress Less, Balance Emotions & Strengthen Your Growing Mind*. Instant Help, 2021.

Rachel Rabkin Peachman and Anna C. Wilson, *When Children Feel Pain from Everyday Aches to Chronic Conditions*. Harvard University Press, 2022.

Michael A. Thompkins, *The Cognitive Behavioral Therapy Workbook*. New Harbinger, 2024.

Heather Turgeon and Julie Wright, *Generation Sleepless: Why Tweens and Teens Aren't Sleeping Enough and How We Can Help Them*. Tarcher, 2022.

Chris van Tullekan, *Ultra-Processed People: Why We Can't Stop Eating Food That Isn't Food*. Norton, 2025.

Internet Sources

Christina Caron, "When Does Anxiety Become a Problem?," *New York Times*, June 23, 2023. www.nytimes.com.

Abigail Fagan, "Why Teens Are Having So Much Less Sex," *Sexual Intelligence* (blog), *Psychology Today*, August 2, 2022. www.psychologytoday.com.

Molly Fisher, "Is It in the Phones?," *New Yorker*, July 7 & 14, 2025. www.newyorker.com.

Abraham Gutman, "Lawsuit over Ultra-Processed Foods Is Tossed," *Philadelphia (PA) Inquirer*, August 26, 2025. www.inquirer.com.

Jarrin Hall, "Students Choose Fast Food for Convenience Despite Health Risks," *The Prospector*, February 5, 2023. https://mshsprospector.org.

Julie Mazziotta and Stephanie Emma Pfeffer, "Weight Loss for Teens Is Controversial: 4 Share How—and Why—They Took Charge of Their Health," *People*, August 29, 2019. https://people.com.

Rob Mentzer, "Teens Talk About How They Maintain Their Mental Health," Wisconsin Public Radio, May 7, 2021. www.wpr.org.

Spencer Plato, "Tommy John Surgeries Are Increasing in Teen Athletes Playing Baseball," Houston Public Media, June 10, 2024. www.houstonpublicmedia.org.

Benjamin Zablotsky et al., "Daily Screen Time Among Teenagers: United States, July 2021–December 2023," Centers for Disease Control and Prevention, 2024. www.cdc.gov.

Organizations and Websites

Centers for Disease Control and Prevention (CDC)
www.cdc.gov
The CDC is the nation's premier public health agency. Its website is full of information and statistics on health concerns relevant to teens: pregnancy, driving, dating violence, vaccination, obesity, and more.

DOZE
www.dozeapp.ca
Learn about a free app designed to provide teens with the tools they need for better sleep. The app was designed by Dr. Colleen Carney, director of the Sleep and Depression Laboratory at Ryerson University in Toronto, Canada. Students who submit a two-week sleep diary can receive feedback and a sleep plan. The app is available via Google Play and the App Store.

Jed Foundation
https://jedfoundation.org
This nonprofit's mission is to help teens and young adults with their mental health. It offers advice and ways to get help for cyberbullying, loneliness, suicide ideation, self-injury, anxiety, depression, and more. It also offers advice for helping a troubled friend.

MedlinePlus
https://medlineplus.gov
MedlinePlus is a good source of health and wellness information for teens that is part of the National Institutes of Health. Find information

and statistics on smoking, underage drinking, illness prevention, sexual health, and many other topics.

National Alliance on Mental Illness (NAMI)
www.nami.org
The NAMI has a special section devoted to kids, teens, and young adults with tips on how to get mental health support. There are tips for talking to friends and parents and information on the role social media plays in mental health. Visitors can find a local chapter and access a twenty-four-hour helpline.

Safe Kids Worldwide
www.safekids.org
An international nonprofit, Safe Kids Worldwide provides information, tips, and resources for the prevention of unintentional injuries to children and teenagers. The website offers videos, as well as information on everything from sports injury prevention to water safety to traffic accidents and falls and burns.

Sleep Cycle
https://sleepcycle.com
Although Sleep Cycle is a paid app, its website offers free content on getting better sleep. For example, there is a nine-question sleep test to evaluate how teens are currently sleeping and information on insomnia, sleep apnea, and other relevant sleep topics.

Start School Later
www.startschoollater.net
Start School Later is an advocacy group for the movement to move school times to make it easier for students to get sufficient sleep. It has more than 165 chapters around the world. Its website has a sleep calculator that helps visitors figure out how much sleep they need and what time they should go to bed, along with success stories and facts about the relationship between school start times and academic success.

Teen Line
https://didihirsch.org/teenline
Trained teenage counselors offer peer-to-peer listening support to other teens who may be struggling with relationship issues, loneliness, and family problems. Find out how to become a teen counselor and download information about dating violence, anxiety, talking about sex, and more.

INDEX

Note: Boldface page numbers indicate illustrations.